STYLING MASCULINITY

STYLING MASCULINITY

Gender, Class, and Inequality
in the Men's Grooming Industry

KRISTEN BARBER

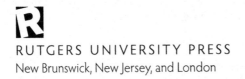

RUTGERS UNIVERSITY PRESS
New Brunswick, New Jersey, and London

Library of Congress Cataloging-in-Publication Data
Names: Barber, Kristen, author.
Title: Styling masculinity : gender, class, and inequality in the men's grooming industry / Kristen Barber.
Description: New Brunswick, New Jersey : Rutgers University Press, 2016. | Includes bibliographical references and index.
Identifiers: LCCN 2015042936| ISBN 9780813565606 (hardcover : alk. paper) | ISBN 9780813565521 (pbk. : alk. paper) | ISBN 9780813565613 (e-book web pdf) | ISBN 9780813572659 (e-book)
Subjects: LCSH: Masculine beauty (Aesthetics) | Grooming for men. | Cosmetics for men. | Beauty shops. | Cosmetics industry. | Sex role.
Classification: LCC HQ1090.27 .B37 2016 | DDC 646.7/044—dc23
LC record available at http://lccn.loc.gov/2015042936

A British Cataloging-in-Publication record for this book is available from the British Library.

Visit our website: http://rutgerspress.rutgers.edu

Manufactured in the United States of America

For Bea

CONTENTS

PREFACE

Brylcreem, a little dab'll do ya,
Brylcreem, you'll look so debonair.
Brylcreem, the gals'll all pursue ya,
They'll love to get their fingers in your hair.
                    —1950s TV jingle for Brylcreem hair pomade

My dad was a stunt pilot. Born in 1925, he began his career crop dusting and was part of the barnstormer era with open cockpits and bi-wing planes. When I was a child I knew him as the center of a group of local airshow performers who traveled the country dazzling audiences of thousands with their death-defying tricks. These were real men. They worked in dirty airplane hangars, and in their younger years some had girlfriends in several cities. I thought back to this group of men as I began my research on men and beauty, especially to my father. I thought about how my brother and I used to play in his relic of a 1950s vibrating exercise machine, an olive green upright mechanism with a wide strap attached to it. The strap wrapped around your waist, hips, or buttocks and was supposed to jiggle the fat off you. I remembered stories of my dad dipping into women's hair dye and moisturizers. One time, preparing for a television interview, he ran a greasy glob of Brylcreem through his hair and down his face. My mom recalls that it was difficult to see him on television since the camera lights created an impossible glare on his slick face. He loyally purchased English Leather cologne from the drugstore, which was known to be a bit more stylish than Brute or Aqua Velva. So, was my dad a metrosexual? By today's standards, not a chance. Yet his participation in the men's grooming market, as limited as it was in the mid- to late-twentieth century, hints that it is a mistake to think of men as nonparticipants in the beauty industry—even those men who lived in a pre-metrosexual era and who we might think of as too masculine to care about their appearances.

My father's bodily repertoire looked much different from that of my youngest brother, who, in 2003 at the age of twelve, carefully lined up his designer colognes along the bathroom mirror—Armani, Abercrombie, Victoria's Secret Very Sexy for Him—and incessantly tossed his styled blond bangs out of his face with an air of finesse. My dad and brother represent snapshots through time of men's long, albeit changing, relationship with beauty. One key distinction between the primpers and preeners of today and those of yesteryear is that men now have access to an abundance of products and services marketed specifically to them. My dad was relegated to the drugstore for the purchase of few men's grooming products. He probably approached a small shelf of shaving cream and cologne nestled near the back of the store. Today, men make up a significant consumer market within the beauty industry, and so corporations that once sold beauty products and services to women are now also appealing to men and their wallets. Department stores like Bloomingdale's have cosmetic counters that carry men's labels, including Lab Series, The Art of Shaving, and Jack Black. Even Target stores stock an array of men's shower gels and hairstyling products. Marketing campaigns aimed at men are attempting with seeming success to intertwine masculine identities with beauty consumption—which is something cosmetic companies accomplished with women only as recently as World War II.[1]

The rise of the metrosexual in the mid-1990s injected the idea of a well-groomed, image-conscious, and brand-obsessed straight man into public discourse. And when I began doctoral work at the University of Southern California, newspaper journalists for the *New York Times* and *Chicago Tribune* were documenting men's forays into nail salons and designer clothing stores.[2] While a plethora of scholarly research had emerged to explore both the oppressive and sometimes liberating aspects of women's different beauty habits, there were few systematic studies attempting to explain what it means for men to participate in similar practices.[3] Popular discourse had also ignored men's long history with beautifying and assumed that men's contemporary participation in fashion and beauty represented the dissolution of gender inequality. Even feminist scholar Susan Bordo, in her book on *The Male Body* in advertising, exclaimed, "I never dreamed that 'equality' would move in the direction of men worrying *more* about their looks rather than women worrying less."[4]

In an effort to move beyond both popular and scholarly assumptions about the meaning of men's beauty, I designed a study that focused on the male clientele of a small women's hair salon in Southern California, Shear Style.[5] This was my first attempt to observe firsthand men's participation in beauty, and I was able to sit down and interview them about how and why they became loyal clients of the salon. These mostly white, well-to-do men paid for a haircut three times the cost of what they could get at the barbershop down the road, and they ventured into an otherwise feminine space with pink walls, cookie platters, flower arrangements, and a majority of women. They made sense of this gender-boundary crossing by focusing on the importance of professional-looking and "stylish" hair, as well as on the friendships they believed they had built with the women stylists. They reinforced classed differences between themselves and working-class white men, who they claimed simply did not care enough about their appearances to patronize such places. Their purchase of commercial beauty services did not result in gender equity, as Bordo might suggest, so much as it reinforced hierarchical differences between men along the lines of race and class.

While this research focused on clients, a group interview with three of the salon's stylists sparked my interest in the labor that supported the men's narratives. I was especially intrigued by the disparities between men's consumer experiences and women's work experiences—since these experiences arise simultaneously. The men at Shear Style, for example, described their stylists as important people in their lives. The women confirmed that they indeed developed affection for some of their clients, but their stories of working on men emphasized the labor involved in cultivating friendly relationships with clients. They knew clients' loyalty—and the size of their tips—hung on their ability to create esteem-building relationships with the men in their chairs. They also complained about the men behind closed doors, exasperated that balding men brought in magazine clippings of well-coiffed celebrities like Brad Pitt as inspirations for their own haircuts.

Men's commercial grooming has flourished since the days my father secretly dipped into my mother's creams and purchased cologne at the drugstore. Men's grooming now constitutes a large, visible subsector of the beauty industry and with it, products for men and new service work opportunities have proliferated. A mainly female workforce of hairstylists, estheticians, nail technicians, and cosmetic counter sales associates mediate men's relationships with beauty. They work tirelessly to sell men products, to educate them on the importance of maintaining and improving their appearances, and to provide them with a particular consumer experience.

Yet these women are missing from scholarly research. As I designed the study for this book, I wanted to know how working with male clients influences the occupational responsibilities, satisfaction, and identities of these women. I asked: How does gender impact the interactions between women beauty workers and their male clients? What is the role of class, sexuality, and race in spaces dedicated to men's grooming, and how do these structures inform client privileges and worker obligations? What do women like about working in these places and working with and on the bodies of men? What would they change? And how do corporations sell beauty to men in the first place?

I explore these questions in this book. Looking closely at two high-service men's salons in Southern California, Adonis and The Executive, I bring men and the women who groom them into the literature on beauty, service work, consumption, and social inequality. I spent time with the women (and the few men) who work in these places, observed the interactions between workers and clients, and interviewed hairstylists, barbers, nail technicians, receptionists, managers, and a massage therapist, esthetician, shoe shiner, and salon owner about working in men's grooming. What I found was a connection between consumption and service work, where women who labor on men's bodies are integral components of men's beauty experiences. I also found that this labor underpins larger corporate marketing strategies, whereby the historically feminized hair salon becomes a masculine place offering masculinizing services and consumer experiences on the shop floor. This book helps to shine light on a growing consumer trend and a new occupational niche—beauty workers who specialize in men's grooming—and is embedded in the historical legacy of men's body projects and the unequal social relations that make these projects possible. While I use a case study of men's salons to discuss the social character and politics of beauty, bodies, and gender relationships, this work has implications for better understanding the complexities and contradictions of work and consumption in the service industry more generally.

ACKNOWLEDGMENTS

Over the years it took me to research and write this book, I relied on the generous feedback and steady encouragement of many people. No book is a solo venture; there are people behind the scenes reading and offering ideas on drafts of chapters and lending an ear when obstacles make research and writing difficult. It is with the enormous support of editors, reviewers, mentors, colleagues, friends, and family that this book is possible.

I owe a special debt of gratitude to the women and men of Adonis and The Executive for allowing me to study their work lives. Securing interviews and conducting observations and surveys are no easy tasks, yet the owners, employees, and clients at these salons welcomed me and made themselves readily available. This project would not exist without their generosity, and to them I am especially grateful.

At Rutgers, I would like to thank project editor, Peter Mickulas, who was a proponent of the book early on. His firm yet gentle push to get on with it helped me move through the final phases of writing and revising. Press reviewers, Karla Erikson and Jamie Mullaney, provided careful readings of the manuscript and advocated for publication. And the work of production editor Carrie Hudak, prepress director Marilyn Campbell, and copy editor Nicole Manganaro, helped to get the book into shape.

The research for this book began at the University of Southern California, where I worked with Michael A. Messner, who has served as a model for doing thoughtful research with an emphasis on how inequality persists and, at times, is undermined by people everyday. Pierrette Hondagneu-Sotelo has also been a wonderful mentor throughout the research and writing process. She has taught me to emphasize the conflict, joy, and humor in the lives of research participants. I would also like to acknowledge Lanita Jacobs and my dissertation writing group: Suzel Bozada-Deas, James McKeever, Evren Savci, and Nicole Willms for their feedback in the early stages of writing up my findings. A special thank-you to colleagues who read drafts of chapters: Tristan Bridges, Catherine Connell, Kirsten Dellinger, Laura Hamilton, and C. J. Pascoe. Timothy J. Haney's enthusiasm for this project buoyed my confidence, and he read excerpts and offered me his opinion when I most needed it. Edward Flores offered his friendship and keen insight throughout this project. Everyone should be as lucky to have such great friends and colleagues.

Many thanks to my colleagues at Southern Illinois University, Carbondale for helping me find time for this undertaking amid a busy schedule of teaching and committee work. I appreciate Christopher Stout for his constant enthusiasm for the book writing process and Kelsy Kretschmer for allowing me to bend her ear when the daily task of moving the project forward became overwhelming. I also had the help of several graduate research assistants who scoured the manuscript for typos, dug around for labor statistics, retrieved literature, and helped to format the manuscript. To Annie Munch, Shiloh Deitz, Megan Rabe, and, especially, Tony Silva and Trisha Crewshaw, thank you.

I would also like to recognize my mother, Elaine Barber. She raised me mostly as a single mother and sacrificed to send me to college. I am grateful that she supported my graduate school career, and I hope I have made her as proud as she makes me.

Thank you to my partner in life, Damien Ricklis. He lived with this project more than anyone else, providing me countless pep talks, feeding and caffeinating me while I wrote, and helping me to celebrate every step along the way. Our two small pugs, Hercules and Lydia, made sure I got out for walks and were there to warm my feet at the end of a long day. I wrote the bulk of this book while pregnant with my daughter, Beatrice, and finalized the manuscript after she was born. In a sense I wrote this book with her. Her small head squeezed up under my ribs while I typed at the coffee shop, and she later played patiently on the living room floor while I lay next to her revising prose on my laptop. Her energy and happiness shaped my attitude in the final phases of the project, and to her I dedicate this book.

STYLING MASCULINITY

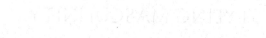

INTRODUCTION

The Style Guy columnist for *Details* then *GQ* magazine, Glenn O'Brien, helps to solve men's "sartorial conundrums" by answering questions about hair loss, offering recommendations for seasonal accessories, and soothing men's worries about using blow dryers.[1] Should men have manicures? "Why not," he writes, "my grandfather used to get manicured at the barbershop, and his nails always looked good." Can men shave their underarms? "More and more guys are shaving areas of their bodies that were once virgin forest. I'm not crazy about the look, but it is preferable to resembling a yeti or a Sasquatch." O'Brien also tries to keep men from making aesthetic mistakes they are sure to regret. For example, should a man with a long "mane" slick back his hair? He retorts, "Have you ever seen a horse covered in pomade? Not a pretty sight. I think the slicked-back look can be quite elegant, but it's not easily carried off."[2]

Addressing grooming dilemmas from around the country, O'Brien works to make beauty A-OK for men. He uses humor and reveals his own beauty regimens—such as shaving his chest—to assure men they are not compromising their masculinity by wanting to look good and shoring up their appearances. Are you a man who wants to trim your eyebrows, get a facial, or shave your balding head? Please, yes, and of course. And, surprise, you are not alone. Going straight to the heart of men's insecurities around their bodies, consumption, and grooming, he paints a picture of a smart, modern man who is successfully moving beyond the prehistoric masculinity of less "elegant," more "yeti" appearing men.[3] O'Brien helps to usher men into contemporary masculine aesthetics, serving as an industry expert in men's styling and a cultural mediator between men's consumer and grooming habits and the meanings or consequences of these habits.

There is a swelling grooming industry that sells and supports men's beauty habits, and it is unlike anything we have seen in the past. Although men have a history of corporeal coiffing, more recent social memory ties beauty to women's culture and to the feminization of bodies. Women in the nineteenth century shared recipes with each other for skin cream, and manufacturers in the 1940s successfully linked lipstick to definitions of good womanhood.[4] Masculinity and beauty, therefore, seem at odds with each other. This is particularly the case for straight men, who are supposed to eschew associations with women and femininity.[5] But with a 2014 Men's Grooming Product sales of almost $6.3 billion,[6] and market research emphasizing men's increasing interest in nail services and pricey haircuts,[7] it is clear that men are spending significant time and money in the larger beauty industry.

What is it that fuels men's interests in and excitement around stylish haircuts and under-eye cream? Some people believe there is a cultural feminization of men in the United States that encourages their entrée into beauty salons and purchase of hair products. "The traditional male is an endangered species," cried *Newsweek* magazine's 2010 September cover. In a sense, this is absolutely correct: something is changing about contemporary masculinities, especially for middle- and upper-middle-class men who might be spending more time on housework than they once did, and who are secondary earners in heterosexual marriages or stay at home to raise their children.[8] These numbers, however, are still small, with slight bumps in statistics underpinning popular assumptions about grand shifts in masculinities and gender relations.[9] Although some men who invest in beautifying products and services indeed see themselves as new, progressive men,[10] the allure of these consumer practices extends to the maintenance of middle-class definitions of what sociologist Raewyn Connell refers to as "hegemonic"—or contextually rewarded—masculinity, by which straight white men are especially advantaged.[11]

Selling men beauty products and services means selling them on the idea that their consumer habits make them men and preserve rather than jeopardize their sexual and class locations. Consider O'Brien, who assures men that they should not doubt the value of a "beauty regimen," and who confidently states, "If trying to look better is girlie, you can call me Mary."[12] Beauty regimens, he suggests, don't have to be emasculating or threatening to men's heterosexual identities—you just have to have the chutzpah (and money) to invest in them. It is not a coincidence that he assumes an audience of professional men who want to look "elegant," or whose financial costs to shore up their appearances might be tax deductible. *GQ*, after all, caters to professional men, publishing columns such as "The GQ Guide to Business Casual."[13] Tucked in its pages are clothing and accessory ensembles with designer names and hefty price tags. "The Man Bag Mans Up," states one editorial. "Get yourself a serious shoulder bag—the kind that no one will mistake for a purse." Recommended? A plaid leather Ally Capellino messenger bag available at Bloomingdale's for $335.[14]

The grooming habits recommended by O'Brien, the men's accessories sold at Bloomingdale's, and the pampering beauty amenities of high-service salons—which emphasize emotional and physical relaxation—are not for all men. Rather, they are integral to a classed gender body project through which well-to-do men come to feel like and identify as well-to-do men. While gay men are popularly associated with feminine cultural markers and practices such as scrupulous style and expensive cosmetics, it is clear these things are being folded into definitions of heterosexual masculinity for men who don't want to look like a Sasquatch. As for the racial and ethnic backgrounds of men consuming style and beauty? This is harder to identify since market research does not report what sort of men are exercising purchasing power in the beauty industry. What we do know, however, is that the everyday barbershop remains an important site for building communities and economies in black neighborhoods[15] but seem to have dwindled in white wealthy neighborhoods,[16] and that white men trade on racial and economic privilege to cross aesthetic gender-boundaries as metrosexuals and hipsters.[17] White bodies and black and brown bodies have different histories, and so the socially informed corporeal adornment of these bodies also looks different. This is not to say that men of color don't have their own history of wanting to look good, but rather that these sorts of practices are associated more with the repudiation of racial and ethnic marginalization than with the preservation of social advantage.[18]

Cultural mediators help men to navigate their relationships with the beauty industry and their identities as consumers. More central than columnists like O'Brien, however, are those people men come into contact with daily who sell and deliver them services and who help them to choose and apply products. Men don't just exfoliate, someone sells them exfoliator and explains its pore-cleansing effects. Men don't just wake up with well-coiffed locks, someone cuts their hair and teaches them how to use sculpting wax to reproduce a hairstyle. In this book, I explore how a class-privileged, heterosexual, masculine consumer is created through inter-actions with beauty service workers. This female-dominated workforce initiates men into beauty culture by providing them the tools to project heteromasculine identities and to think of themselves as professional men precisely because of their participation in the beauty industry.

Through a study of high-service men's salons in Southern California, Adonis and The Executive,[19] I explain how women beauty workers come to bear the burden of grooming men. Doing so, I take a ground-up approach to explaining the phenomenon of the male beauty consumer: exploring in-depth two field sites to interrogate larger questions around how the grooming industry does not just generate products and services specifically for men, but also creates a middle-class, heteromasculine, and often white consumer in the process. As beauty industry corporations, Adonis and The Executive use assorted strategies to cultivate a masculine and masculinizing consumer experience. The spaces—including architectural detail, décor, and amenities—and the salons' institutionalized "masculine verbiage," for example, reflect the power of harnessing the cultural symbolic order to cultivate brand images and encourage clients' engagement with structures of gender, heterosexuality, race, and class. And service employees like the women at these salons are incorporated into the commercial environment and consumer experience, supporting clients' identities and privileges on the shop floor.

The worker-client interaction is crucial in creating a willing male beauty consumer. Focusing on how these interactions play out in high-service men's salons, this book reveals the social relations and inequalities in recod-ing beauty for men. It is women who are disproportionately responsible for mediating men's relationships with beauty spaces, products, and services. They are organizationally commodified and interpersonally objectified to create an ego-enhancing beauty experience for the salons' male clientele. By focusing on the narratives of the women and the few men who work at Adonis and The Executive, I find that these workers uphold the mas-culinizing brand image of the salons while also negotiating the meaning of their labor. The demands made on women's gendered identities, emo-tions, appearances, and bodily labor both support a masculine beauty con-sumer and allow the women to etch out a sense of professionalism and job satisfaction. *Styling Masculinity* provides insight into the labor processes of women workers who wrestle organizational demands that set them up as gendered persons first and skilled workers second.

I bring together the sociology of consumption with the sociology of service work to show that as employees are increasingly incorporated into the commercial environment, their responsibilities shift to support organizational branding goals and consumer experiences. As such, this book is a study in the sociology of bodies, emotions, spaces, and symbolic constructions of sameness and difference; and drawing from feminist theories in these areas and responding to scholarly calls to link micro-analyses to larger structures, I add to and revise current insights from the gender, work, and consumption literature. At Adonis and The Executive, I find that the workers and consumers are produced through the salons' branding efforts, women's creation of valued work identities, and men's investment in their symbolic and structural privilege. Instructions, pratices, and material goods come together to shape the relationships and professional status of these men and women. Gender in the marketplace, I argue, is not only best understood through an intersectional perspective that considers other locations like race and class, but is also a tangible cultural tool corporations use to encourage consumers to cross social boundaries while making this boundary crossing a status-enhancing practice. Engaging popular frames of postfeminism, the data in this book encourage us to think more critically about how gender and class locations, and seemingly benign experiences, are key to identity formation and often uneven social relations.

WHERE IS THE BEAUTIFUL MAN?

Research on beauty tends to focus on women and overlooks the ways men primp their bodies to carve out social identities and access social rewards. Scholarly and public criticism of beauty norms highlight women's complicated relationships with their appearances. Conventional feminine beauty expectations are thin, white, and unattainable for most without the help of Photoshop, and they create a sort of bodily panopticon by which women evaluate their bodies, compare themselves to others, and come to invest a great deal of time, energy, and money in their appearances.[20] In her book *The Beauty Myth*, Naomi Wolf argues that women could be doing more important things than aestheticizing, and that beauty as an all-consuming body project ultimately subordinates women.[21] Around the world and throughout time different cultural ideologies and rituals have controlled women's bodies and thus constrained their participation in public and political life.

This critical feminist perspective on beauty sheds light on the material effects of the sex/gender system. More recently, however, scholars have argued that conceptualizing women's beauty routines as solely oppressive limits our understanding of the role bodies play in reimagining power and dominance. It ignores how beauty routines help women to forge proud identities and personal friendships and are experienced by women as fun and pleasurable. Depending on their race, class, and sexual orientation, women have different relationships to beauty,[22] and bodily repertoires and styles sort women into racialized and classed hierarchies, allowing them to "do difference."[23] Miliann Kang's research on Korean nail salons, for instance, finds that black women frequent salons where workers emphasize feelings of racial equality and create elaborate nail designs.[24] Middle-class white women more often invest in conservative nail colors and prefer technicians to pamper them emotionally, which upholds unquestioned racial privilege, the subordination of immigrant women, and an aesthetic that separates them from racial "others."

Feminist theories on gender and beauty have expanded to take seriously women's feelings of pleasure in modifying their bodies. Beauty routines put women in touch with other women so they might create supportive communities with each other at the beauty shop or while doing each other's hair at the kitchen table.[25] And some women enjoy the perks that come with meeting, diverting from, or reimagining beauty norms.[26] Beauty is not an all or nothing practice. It is a multifaceted social ritual that allows women to access class privileges, to resist racial oppression, and to feel strong, healthy, and confident.[27] Women's subjectivities cannot be reduced to the internalization of the male gaze. It is not always about men—feelings of pleasure matter; hierarchies among women matter; micro-aggressions that challenge the status quo matter. Women are continually redefining the symbolic order where the body is otherwise "directly involved in a political field" of power and where "power relations have an immediate hold upon it."[28]

Gender scholarship has focused on the importance of beauty in women's lives and the meaning of beauty norms vis-à-vis men's dominance, but it has also taken for granted beauty as particular to women. We might even think that "grooming" and "handsome" are more appropriate terms to describe men, and that "beauty"—as it is associated with vanity and scrupulous aestheticizing—describes only women. Men's relationships to beauty, from this perspective, can be understood only as evaluators of women's heterofeminine appearances and as beneficiaries of the subordinating effects of beauty practices. It is important to take seriously men's objectification of and entitlement to women's bodies, since these place women at risk of stereotyping, discrimination, and sexual assault.[29] Yet this perspective also rests squarely on assumptions of heterosexuality and reproduces inadequate Cartesian philosophies on the separation of mind and body.[30] Patriarchal ideologies characterize men as somehow disembodied, rational beings and reduce women to the whims of their bodies and emotions. Men do, women are. But men too are embodied and, as I argue here, they have a complicated relationship with beauty and their bodies as sites of privilege, power, and pleasure.

Scholars have discussed the fetishized male form in Ancient Rome and the decorated Regency dandy,[31] but today's beautiful man has largely escaped empirical investigation. Contemporary research on men's bodies looks at men's involvement in domestic and sexual assault, the building of muscle, and dominating other men on the football field and in the locker room.[32] These are important foci for theorizing men's bodies as sources of power and for revealing that trying to live up to expectations of hegemonic masculinity can result in costs,[33] like incurring physical injuries and missing out on close intimate relationships with others. This research considers the more obvious ways men attempt to approximate hegemonically masculine bodies via strength, aggression, and other displays of physical dominance—creating the impression that men's bodies are worth scholarly attention only when they are hypermasculine. Some studies, like those on drag queens, indeed look at the transgressive male body,[34] but also miss out on how men's careful clothing decisions and scrupulous hair management can create culturally valorized or rewarded masculinities. Building muscle and exerting strength are not the only ways to fashion a dominant, privileged male body. It is also a consumer project buoyed by seemingly feminizing practices and a female-dominated workforce.

By emphasizing an analysis of privilege, I answer the question: Why should we care about the beautiful and beautifying man? As long as men's bodies are visible only in masculine institutions, we risk overlooking how men reproduce power through seemingly subversive activities. The sex/gender system affects men and women differently, and so we cannot simply apply the lessons learned from studying women to understand men and beauty. In my earlier research, I found that a class-privileged and largely white group of men invest in stylish haircuts as a distinguishing practice, similar to women.[35] But at the same time they set themselves apart from and above their working-class counterparts, these men also shunned femininity.[36] I dig deeper here and argue that more empirical and theoretical work is necessary to understand men's complex relationships with the beauty industry and the social implications of these relationships. Applying feminist theories on the gender order, I consider the ways cultural assumptions about masculinity, class and racial privilege, and heterosexual identities are reflected in and reproduced via the interaction of social structures, organizational cultures, and worker-client engagements.

THEORIZING THE LABOR OF CONSUMPTION

Women workers are essential to the culture of producing male beauty. When I began research for this book, I was interested in male beauty consumers. The workers were there, but they were in the background. Building on my previous research, which looks at how men make sense of crossing gender boundaries into a women's hair salon, I wanted to better understand how men weave narratives of masculinity in ways that reimagine beauty services and spaces. The gender of culture and consumption: that was my focus. But as I gained entrée into Adonis and The Executive, it became clear that looking exclusively at the consumer overshadowed the work involved in creating male beauty consumers. So I shifted my attention to the labor of women who support men in these salons. Bringing together feminist scholarship on the cultural symbolic order with that on class, gender, and race as performances and interactions, I theorize the gender of beauty work in creating a new consumer niche and a privileged manhood in a space and through practices popularly associated with women.

Feminist work on the cultural symbolic order highlights the importance of artifacts. People generally presume artifacts are things we make, but we collectively craft more than objects. The material world also includes cultural norms, social processes, ideologies, and languages. Getting one's hair cut and styled at a salon produces a hairdo, which is a tangible cultural artifact that reflects gendered institutions and moments in history: the beehive; the Farrah Fawcett; the flattop. Yet the processes of seeking out and getting or giving a haircut similarly reveal cultural norms that are the building blocks of social structures. The class-privileged salon client, for example, is created and re-created at the point of purchase as consumer experiences are carefully cultivated by management, informed by popular local customs, and continually produced and manipulated within shop floor interactions. These processes generate experiences people often take for granted; for example, to the upper-middle class it makes sense salon workers would offer men imported beer and women hot tea or a glass of champagne. But organizations draw on particular assumptions about masculinity when providing men beer and instructing female employees to fetch the beer. When women receptionists or stylists hand men beer, they engage in both an economic and gendered (and sometimes racially salient) service interaction. When men drink their beer, they associate themselves with a symbolic culture of manhood.

From a sociological standpoint, cultural objects cannot be understood in isolation from people's engagement with them. This characterizes the study of symbolic interaction, by which we jointly create and relate to the social world.[37] By taking people instead of objects as the unit of analysis, we can see how people resist and remake meaningful frames attached to things. It is also important to consider the institutional and interpersonal contexts in which people engage the material world. Beer alone does not make the man. It is the act of swigging beer and being served by a woman that informs gendered identities and relationships in that moment. The idea that objects have static meanings and monolithic implications for the people who use them limits our understanding of how power operates through the material world. Considering how people engage objects, processes, and ideologies, and how they collectively shape the meaning of these things, requires bringing together cultural analysis with interactionist theories that are sensitive to social structure. This allows us to see how gendered objects and gendered people are manufactured and manipulated as we come together to make sense of and claim our places in the world.

Conceptualizing gender—as well as race, class, and sexuality—as something that is accomplished everyday highlights the contextual character of social status and identities, as well as the ways gender ideologies are produced through embodied exchanges.[38] Of course people can do gender in ways that undermine systems of inequality, but it is difficult to realize the plasticity of gender when we hold others accountable for meeting certain expectations. Men are therefore not created so much when they purchase styling wax or a "MANicure" but as they negotiate the gendered meanings of hairstyling products when chatting with their stylists or their friends and families.

Work was once central to identification, especially for men, but today consumer habits heavily shape the social identities of people in the Global North,[39] as well as how we negotiate membership to different groups and to economic and political systems. George Ritzer calls for sociology to take seriously the importance of consumption in American life, noting that a "strong case could be made that studies of the mall and its customers would tell us at least as much, and probably more, about the larger society than studies of the factory and its workers."[40] He laments that sociology has placed inordinate focus on the production of goods while ignoring the consumption of goods. Here, I advocate an approach that we cannot fully understand the social processes of consumption without taking into account labor processes. Consumption and labor act in tandem to produce our economic life, social hierarchies, and everyday identities. A focus on consumption that ignores labor reproduces the impression that these things emerge and operate separately. And the reverse is true in much of the work and occupations literature: consumption is often overlooked.[41] But what happens when we bring the study of consumption and labor together? How might we come to understand consumer goods and services as products of interactions between customers and workers? And what does this mean for social relations of power?

To answer these questions, I argue that we need to retheorize consumption through the lens of labor and vice versa. A service economy, after all, increases chances for face-to-face interactions, especially in luxury spaces where customers expect personalized service and deferential workers.[42] As recent work on aesthetic labor shows, the service employee is increasingly part of the consumer experience.[43] Corporations hire people who look the brand, with luxury retail stores preferring white, middle-class employees who are also consumers of the brands they sell. These workers signal just who corporations envision their customers to be: similarly white and middle class. Consumers are supposed to see themselves reflected in the worker

(I talk more about this in chapter 3), and this logic has implications for inequalities in service work. Exploring what this sort of labor means for the employee is helpful in unpacking the new demands corporations make on workers. Still, scholars theorizing aesthetic labor often leave out an analysis of the consumer, other than to suggest they ideally relate to the employees with whom they come in contact.[44]

If we think of the beauty industry solely in terms of product consumption or manufacturing and marketing, then we fail to see how people create the meaning of beauty during their interactions with others on the shop floor. From this perspective, the social and cultural significance of a haircut is just as much in the process of getting or giving that haircut as it is in the resulting hairdo. I look at how the labor of women beauty workers involved in the manipulation of men's bodies is central to creating a heteromasculine, middle-class, and often white brand image and consumer experience at men's salons. By considering how women negotiate the demands this labor places on their gender and sexual identities, emotions, and bodies, I build on existing theories of work—including aesthetic labor and "feeling rules"[45]—to understand how the worker and the consumer are simultaneously created via interactive processes surrounding material and commercial culture.

THE SITES AND THE STUDY

Southern California is a major hub for beauty. It is known as the cosmetic surgery capital of the United States and is home to glamorous movie stars like Angelina Jolie and Brad Pitt. People are fascinated by the wealth and consumer culture of the region, with viewers popularizing reality television shows like *The Real Housewives of Orange County*, *Botched*, and *#Rich Kids of Beverly Hills*. Fashion and beauty trends emerge here before spreading across the country and seeping into the aesthetic milieus of rural American high schools and college campuses. The area is replete with cosmetic surgeons, luxury hair and nail salons, designer boutiques, MAC cosmetic stores, cutting-edge fitness gyms, and specialty shops offering eyebrow threading, eyelash extensions, spray tans, and laser cellulite treatments. If you're lucky, you might run into a celebrity or two shopping at Gucci or Prada on Rodeo Drive. Working out at my local gym was always a lesson in corporeal aesthetics, with women decked out in push-up bras, full makeup, and delicate jewelry while whisking away on the elliptic machines and men with spray tans and fresh hair plugs lingering around the weight room mirrors.

With an emphasis on beauty culture and conspicuous consumption, and a history of self-creation, Southern California is an ideal location for the study of men's grooming. Southern California is a postmodern urban area where commodity fetishism and over-the-top leisure proliferate. And there is a saga of selfhood imagined in its urban terrain, as migrant populations have made and remade themselves and the cities in which they live. In a country where talking about class and race can be controversial and even get people into trouble, we turn to gendered bodies as landscapes for constructing and contesting selves in these spaces. This sociohistorical context has created a robust beauty industry that supports aestheticizing consumer practices and requires a bounty of beauty providers, whose numbers total 7,340 in the Los Angeles area.[46]

At the same time it is a mecca for commercial aestheticizing, Southern California is not unique in its growth of a men's beauty market. I anticipate some readers will ask: What can a study of men's beauty in Southern California teach us about men's relationships to their bodies and consumer practices—and about beauty work—in other places? While you might be hard-pressed to find a hair salon dedicated to men in small town America, men's grooming exists on both a national and global scale. The privileged consumer experience, including that at high-service salons, thrives in the Global North, where conspicuous consumption has become a way of life. The United States, Europe, Australia, and some parts of Asia have moved from an era of production to that of consumption, whereby the construction of the self is located in consumer culture. In the United States, Southern California is not a special case in terms of men's beauty practices and spaces, but is instead an example of the classed and urban phenomenon of men's salons. High-service men's salons like the ones in this book are popping up across the country, from Seattle and Dallas to Charlotte and Boston; and journalists document the increasing production of men's cosmetics and fashion. I use industry statistics in the next chapter to show that men's beauty is a growing market with a rise in sales over the last ten years, even during the 2007–2009 Great Recession. These data set the foundation for my findings: instead of being a fleeting trend or an issue particular to Southern California, there are larger shifting norms around middle- and upper-middle-class masculinities and men's consumption, and around the responsibilities and experiences of beauty workers.

In this book, I examine men's beauty consumption in a growing national consumer landscape by using men's salons as an empirical case. When I explain my research to people, they often ask, "What is a *men's* salon, exactly?" This is precisely the question guiding this book. I explore here what men's salons look like, how they are produced, and what they mean for the people who spend time there. As a qualitative sociologist, I am interested in meanings as they are constructed through people's face-to-face exchanges and how the organizations in which these exchanges are embedded shape relationships between groups of people, identity building processes, and the reproduction and reimagining of cultural norms. I often take this question quite literally, though, answering that men's salons are just that: salons dedicated to the primping and preening of men. High-end men's salons offer an array of services, including haircuts, hair coloring, manicures, pedicures, facials, and sometimes massages and body waxing. And they market these services directly to men.

To more accurately explain what a men's salon is means delving into sociological understandings of gender as something that is produced rather than something that is static and that we inherently possess. Men's salons are not just men's salons because they appeal to and serve a male clientele. As sociologist Dana Britton notes, "To say that organizations are *inherently* gendered implies that they have been defined, conceptualized, and structured in terms of a distinction between masculinity and femininity, and presume and will thus inevitably reproduce gendered differences."[47] Organizations may indeed be gendered, but this should not be presumed.[48] If we consider instead the everyday creation of meaning, then we can see just how places, processes, and people come to be gendered. So when looking at Adonis and The Executive, I ask: How do men's salons become masculine spaces? What sort of organizational and interpersonal processes produce men in these spaces? What does this production mean for the women and men who work there, for clients' relationships to larger cultural definitions of masculinity, and for norms regulating men and women's relationships? That is, what are the social relations underpinning the production and growth of a new men's market?

I conducted field observations at Adonis and The Executive. These salons are decked out in solid woods, clean lines, leather chairs, and charge upward of $39 for a haircut—more than three times the usual $12 barber-shop or chain salon haircut. Of course, men could spend even more money at trendy unisex salons in West Hollywood or Beverly Hills. Adonis and The Executive keep haircuts affordable for middle-class men at the same time they weed out blue-collar men who might scoff at the monetary and personal investment in vanity, and who might instead define a weathered body as a marker of masculinity.[49] Carefully coiffed hair helps professional men navigate white-collar expectations of embodiment—signaling competence and control—and to distinguish themselves from poor and working-class men; and for white men, from men of color.[50] Adonis and The Executive appeal to well-to-do white men who are moving up from the everyday barbershop, who are too elitist for chain stores like Supercuts, or who are not comfortable at more hoity-toity unisex salons.

I began this study in the winter of 2009, when a research fellowship allowed me to concentrate on data collection. I chose to focus on high-service men's salons because they are places where men seek both a "superior" product and a particularly gendered and classed experience that is wrapped up with luxurious spaces and pampering services. While men might suggest they are there for the haircut, their motivations are much more complicated than this; and the salons, as corporate organizations, carefully orchestrate every aspect of men's consumer experiences. I relied on the methods of in-depth interviewing and ethnographic observations for collecting data on how meanings around men's beauty and consumer identities are shaped by their interactions with a largely female workforce of beauty providers. I supplemented these data with analyses of the salons' corporate websites, customer surveys at The Executive, and online customer reviews of fifteen different men's salons in Southern California.

Adonis was the first salon at which I gained permission to research. Before this, salon managers and owners were nervous that my presence might make clients feel self-conscious about pursuing high-service beauty. When I approached Tyler, the owner of Adonis, about studying his salon, he appeared delighted that I was interested in what he was doing with men's grooming. Through a bit of backdoor bragging, he explained that journalists are "always writing articles on us." He liked the public exposure and, while he said he did not have the time to participate in an interview himself, agreed to let me observe workers and clients and to interview his employees. Veronica, owner of The Executive, also immediately granted me permission to study her salon. She is a supporter of higher education and appreciates the value of research and academic interest in businesses. Ethnographers talk about the importance of deeply immersing themselves into their field sites, gaining access to all corners of a space and to the behind-the-scenes interactions during which participants make decisions about organizational goals and, in my case, gossip about clients and coworkers. However, while Tyler and Veronica graciously allowed me to come back to their salons time and time again to study the spaces, worker-client interactions, and marketing strategies, I never became a real insider.

During my earlier research in salons, I quickly discovered how difficult it is to become a participant observer in workplaces. Without two years of training and a cosmetology or barber license, I could not work alongside the stylists and nail technicians. Years ago, I offered to sweep up hair and shampoo clients at a women's salon in exchange for studying their site; stylists retorted that I had to have 1,600 hours of cosmetology training to do so and that those jobs belong to apprentices. I realized I had insulted the stylists by suggesting that I could do these jobs without their training. So for the nine months I studied Adonis and The Executive, I became a regular fixture without becoming a true insider. I built casual relationships with many of the women and men who worked at the salons, and this certainly aided in our familiarity and the building of more mutual relationships where they asked about my life and probed into my research intentions. And while I could ask them what happened in the break rooms of the salons, I was never allowed back there.[51]

The bulk of my data come from interviews I conducted with the hairstylists, barbers, nail technicians, estheticians, receptionists, and managers at both Adonis and The Executive. Adonis also employed a massage therapist. And while Tyler did not do a formal interview with me, Veronica sat down with me on multiple occasions to answer my questions about her short-term and long-term goals for the salon, as well as her hiring and training practices and the philosophies guiding her approach to client care. Although not a beauty worker per se, Antonio, a shoe shiner and sometime janitor at The Executive, spoke with me about what the salon, the clients, and the men's grooming industry looked like from his perspective. A Mexican immigrant who had worked at The Executive for nine years when I spoke with him, Antonio occupied a unique position on the margins of the salon, and his interview helped to highlight the racialization of informal work requirements such as emotionally caring for clients. I also include an interview with Corey, the owner and stylist of a third men's salon in the area, and the only gay stylist in my study. His interview gave me insight into the interpersonal work involved in initiating men into beauty. In total, the experiences and opinions of thirty-six beauty providers working in the men's grooming industry are represented in this book.

Speaking with these women and men allowed me to understand how their bodies and emotions are commercialized and consumed to produce male beauty consumers, as well as how they reimagined their labor to create meaningful identities and negotiate their social statuses. I also talked with clients who could describe their salon experiences and explain their relationships with the salons' beauty providers. Comparing and contrasting the workers' narratives with those of their clients' helped me to better dissect the complex and often contradictory nature of social relationships—as people with different locations and interests come together at these salons in the pursuit of ostensibly the same thing: a great haircut or well-manicured hand.

As I discuss in the methodological appendix, the economic recession together with clients' class and race privileges led the salons' owners to consider clients both precious and vulnerable. Men have plenty of options for hair care, and so Tyler and Veronica did not want my interview solicitation to mar the luxurious experience they worked so hard to provide men, and which they believe is a large reason men came back to their salons. Tyler refused to let me interact much with his clients; I could not interview them and he wanted me to avoid contact with them as much as possible while I observed the salon. Veronica, on the other hand, conceded to a quick customer survey, at the bottom of which I requested participants for follow-up interviews. From these surveys, I gathered interviews with twelve clients of The Executive, many of which took place on the phone as the men squeezed me into their busy work and family lives.[52] I also did an interview with Noah, a friend of mine who was a client at Adonis, and Amit, who frequented a competing men's salon in the area.

Adonis and The Executive are racialized spaces that draw from popular U.S. conceptions of white professional-class masculinity to create a particular commercial experience for their clients. Although they employ Asian and Latino beauty workers and serve Asian, Latino, Middle-Eastern clients, both salons take whiteness for granted. As I will discuss later, displaying magazines like *Golf* and *GQ*, rather than *Ebony* or *Latino*, mark the salons as for white men. Class and gender are salient in Adonis and The Executive's marketing strategies, but whiteness too is embedded in the culture of men's beauty, even if it sits below the surface and reveals itself partly in what or who is *not* present at the salons—black stylists or barbers who specialize in clipper cuts, for instance. This whiteness reflects the sort of masculinity for sale at the salon, and so it is no surprise then that the salons' clients are mostly white (see appendix B).

Peppered throughout this book is supplemental data I gathered from the sixty-nine customer surveys I collected at The Executive, and from content analyses of both the salons' websites and Yelp.com reviews of fifteen local men's salons. Gathering this extra information was a great lesson for me in the necessity of going online for data,[53] and in the fruitfulness of methodological creativity. Customer surveys helped me to get an idea of who exactly goes to The Executive, as well as which services they purchase, where they previously went for their haircuts or mani-pedis, and what they see as the major draws and downsides of the salon. I found that many of the men previously patronized barbershops and women's salons—avoiding low-cost chain salons like Supercuts—and that few of them reported purchasing bodyscaping services like back or "bikini" waxing.

My foray into online data collection was quite accidental. It resulted from the need to find field sites in a sprawling metropolis, the barriers I faced soliciting interviews with the salons' clients, and taking seriously what participants told me about being online—they read, interpret, and referred to clients' online reviews. I found the relationships between the salons, clients, and stylists were forged online as well as on the shop floor. The corporate websites, for example, allowed me to better understand how Adonis and The Executive created masculine brand images and made promises to potential clients before men set foot inside the salons. Online customer reviews of various Southern California men's salons revealed how men negotiate and project public masculine identities in light of their commercial beauty habits and assisted the salons' efforts to craft masculinized definitions of beauty.[54]

ORGANIZATION OF THE BOOK

In chapter 1, I detail the history of men's grooming with a focus on the politics of men's corporeal adornment and on the corporate struggles to make beauty synonymous with masculinity. From courtiers in powdered wigs and pink-gloved dandies to Jesus hair hippies and brand-obsessed metrosexuals, men have long groomed to establish their social locations. This history with fashion and beauty sets the stage for today's man of consumption. I also outline the development and evolution of the larger beauty industry, which was begun by women who concocted creams in their kitchens but proliferated by men with the education, social networks, and financial means to commercialize beauty. Immigrant women and women of color, including Madame C. J. Walker and Florence Nightingale Graham, used their knowledge of beauty culture as a vehicle to pull themselves out of poverty and to forge livelihoods at a time when they had few paths to financial independence. Men seized many of these businesses to create the mass production and market-driven beauty industry we know today, but women remained the bulk of beauty service providers. To more broadly situate the findings in this book, I end this chapter with a detailed description of the growing contemporary U.S. men's grooming industry. I draw from market statistics and popular commercial examples to demonstrate the swelling of both men's product sales and men's purchase of hair and nail services. From Los Angeles to Charlotte, it is clear beauty is being reimagined and sold to men.

The historical trends in men's beauty consumption play out in chapter 2, which centers on the recoding of beauty spaces, products, and services to masculinize a historically feminized institution: the hair salon. The corporate inclusion of "masculine verbiage," for example, helps to socialize men into beauty regimens. "Highlights" become "manlights" and "hair coloring" becomes "color camo." Conventional notions of men and masculinity, as well as cultural markers of race and class privilege, inform the layout, décor, and amenities at Adonis and The Executive, enabling clients' engagement with high-status white masculinity. These salons differ, however, in that Adonis channels a youthful guy culture through the incorporation of video game consoles and The Executive signals a more conservative, nostalgic American manhood via reproduction barber chairs and sandalwood-scented candles. Yet it is the women working at these salons who initiate men into the beauty industry. They help the men navigate salon etiquette, fetch them beer, and introduce them to masculine and masculinizing beauty terminology. I discuss how a *specter of homosociality* operates at the salons, whereby men ignore the omnipresence of women and perceive the salons as like men-only gentlemen's clubs—places appropriate for high-status white men like themselves. At the same time, it is the presence of deferential, consumable women workers that provides them the opportunity to manufacture identities as privileged men.

Chapter 3 introduces the concept of *heterosexual aesthetic labor*, whereby the salons uphold heteromasculine brand images by hiring, developing, and mobilizing the identities of straight, conventionally feminine-looking women. These women serve as commercial tools for the salons and as identity resources by which clients can project heterosexual identities during their haircuts or manis and pedis. This highlights the contextual, temporal, and interactional character of gender and sexuality. While the men working at Adonis and The Executive do not perform heterosexual aesthetic labor in the same way as their female coworkers, they nonetheless have to appear straight so as not to threaten clients' masculinity when having their hair coiffed by another man. I discuss how The Executive, which is particularly invested in creating a classed, gendered brand, institutes professional dress codes and hires college-educated women to support the identities and privileges of a largely white-collar male clientele. These women are caught between their professionalizing desires and the objectifying nature of heterosexual aesthetic labor. I consider how the women use professionalizing discourses and protocols to negotiate this tension, as well as how their abilities to resist the heterosexualizing constraints of their work is limited by the link between heterofeminine identities and the fiscal success of both salons and workers.

Beauty work literature has established the role emotional labor plays in providing an especially white, middle-class consumer experience at salons.[55] This scholarship, however, focuses on interactions between women beauty providers and women customers, overlooking how gender might differently shape this labor when women work on the bodies of men and when men are themselves beauty workers. Chapter 4 explores how systems of gender and heterosexuality impact the feeling rules by which workers at the men's salons end up doing "hairapy." They come to see themselves as "other women" who provide their clients with important confidential friendships;

male stylists, on the other hand, forge "guy time" with clients by both talk-ing clients through their troubles and participating in the collective objecti-fication of women. I highlight moments when the racialization of gendered emotions rises to the forefront of care work in these salons, especially as they play out during interactions between the mainly white clientele and Antonio, The Executive's Mexican immigrant shoe shiner. Elaborating on the notion of feeling rules, which guide emotional expressions and perfor-mances in organizations, and building on Miliann Kang's "bodily labor,"[56] I argue that the beauty workers in this study operate by different *touching rules* when grooming men. These rules help to explain how socially and con-textually specific norms enable and constrain who can touch clients, how so, under what conditions, and how workers are supposed to feel about this touch. Instead of seeing talk and touch as mutually exclusive yet operating simultaneously in beauty work, I am interested in those moments when masculinizing emotional labor is a function of touch. I discuss what all of this means for the commercialization of workers' bodies and emotions, and I unpack how the women create meaningful identities as hairapists and con-sequently pillar gender differences between men and women.

Chapter 5 focuses on the ways these women make sense of their deci-sions to work in salons that are dedicated to men and in jobs that require constant, and often intimate, contact with men. I discuss how the women evoke different *occupational choice narratives*, depending on whether they work solely with men or also part time in a women's salon, and how they forge particular gender identities in the process. Women working in men's salons pick up corporate rhetoric and behaviors to evoke discourses of sameness and difference that ultimately shape their gender identities. Working for a men's salon organized around the careful cultivation and propping up of masculinity, women at The Executive align themselves with their high-status clients by casting themselves as "tomboys" and "men's women." They trade on misogyny to deploy sexist discourses that educe stereotypes about other women, repudiate femininity, and mark themselves as exceptional women. Women at Adonis tend to also work part time at Bonita, a sister salon serving mostly women. These beauty workers display a sense of appreciation for women's culture, the relationships they build with other women, the different occupational skills they sharpen, and the oppor-tunities for work variation at each salon. Working on both men and women creates space for appreciating multiple femininities, while women at The

Executive end up subordinating other women and reinforcing hierarchal gender relations that devalue femininity.

In the concluding chapter, I reiterate how it is that Adonis and The Executive are situated historically in industry efforts to masculinize men's beauty consumption and what they can teach us about the reproduction of social distinction during presumably gender-progressive commercial practices. As the men's grooming market grows, spaces like men's salons, "for men" beauty products, and professional services popularly associated with women and femininity are being institutionally reimagined, recoded, and reorganized. This reorganization affects a largely female workforce that bears the daily responsibility of making beauty not only palatable to, but also status enhancing for already privileged men. Popular rhetoric suggests men's participation in the beauty industry reflects a closing gender gap, with men becoming more like women. Their consumer experiences, however, take place at salons invested in upholding men's performances of privileged heteromasculinity, and which identify and capitalize on unequal class and gender relationships. Important, though, are the liberating and organizing possibilities of beauty work and corporate policy changes that might create a less exploitive work environment for women beauty workers. I stress the significance of women's abilities to negotiate and remake the meaning of their commercialized identities, feelings, and bodies within the confines of their particularly gendered and classed jobs and workplaces. The story of men who consume beauty cannot be told without considering the women who groom them.

1 · MEN AND BEAUTY

The Historical Expansion of an Industry

The metrosexual burst into popular discussions of men's bodies in 1994. British journalist Mark Simpson coined the term in an effort to capture what he saw as a new heterosexual masculinity, one rooted in consumption and vanity. He suggested that it is not just women whose gender identities are cultivated through the production of a beautiful self, but rather that there is a growing consciousness among especially straight, class-privileged men to the pleasures of dabbling in cosmetics and shopping, and in showing off their corporeal assets. Soccer star David Beckham has become the poster boy for metrosexuality. He is at the same time Emporio Armani underwear model, retired soccer star, father of four, and husband to Victoria Beckham, the popstar famously known as Posh Spice. In an opinion piece for CNN.com, journalist Ellis Cashmore noted that Beckham "wore a sarong, a headscarf, nail varnish, adorned his body with tattoos and changes his expertly coiffured hair-do practically every week . . . And yet his masculinity was never in doubt."[1] Olympic swimmer and ladies' dude Ryan Loctche happily admits to spending four to five hours at a time manscaping, shaving his entire body with a hefty, gold-plated razor that looks as if it came out of Liberace's medicine cabinet.[2] At the same time Simpson captures the growing trend of marketing men's bodies and products, though, he also gives the misimpression that men's interest in fashion and beauty is a recent phenomenon.

Men have long fretted over their appearances and gone to great lengths to cultivate their embodiments. Julius Caesar, for instance, wore his signature ceremonial wreath to hide the fact that he was balding. Roman men often kept themselves clean-shaven, stopping in the public square where a barber was on hand to whip the stubble from their chins.[3] Hannibal, a Carthaginian commander who defeated the Romans, waged war while wearing a wig. He also "kept a second one on hand for social occasions."[4] Hair and the lack thereof is just one aspect of embodiment that has long triggered anxiety and self-consciousness in men. And while Western ideological attachment to individualism suggests men's body projects grow out of and reflect personal internal self-doubt, these tensions are connected to larger cultural expectations of masculine embodiments and the organization of social relations.

We tend to think men's participation in beauty brings them closer to women; yet class and race have significantly shaped men's grooming habits and the meanings of their embodiments throughout history. Today, white men who work construction may tout their weathered skin as a symbol of "real" laborious masculinity,[5] and professional-class white men seek out stylish haircuts that distinguish them from and above working-class masculinity.[6] The growing consumer culture has created new means by which men can purchase and groom their way into status groups, aligning themselves with particular class, racial, gender, and sexual locations. So although well-to-do men have long fussed over their appearances, what Simpson captures are the ways masculinity is now marketed back to men in a commercialized, post-industrial U.S. and Western Europe.

Men's consumer participation in the beauty industry is part of the ongoing story of men's historical treatment of their bodies and emerges from manufacturers' struggles to make beauty consumption synonymous with men's identities. While beauty entrepreneurs successfully tied cosmetics to the appropriation of elite femininity in the early twentieth century,[7] folding beauty services and products into culturally valorized expressions of masculinity is a more recent accomplishment. As we consider the beauty industry's evolution to include men as a major consumer sector, it is important to understand men's historical relationship with fashion and beauty, how the male beauty consumer has come to be, what men's spending habits look like, what ideologies encourage these habits, and who exactly is on the frontlines to support men's commercial grooming practices.

MEN'S FASHION AND BEAUTY

Class Status and Racial Politics

Fashion and beauty have not always served to distinguish men from women as much as they have been symbols of class. In ancient Greece, Rome, and Egypt, draped and fitted clothing marked differences between privileged and laboring classes; and in Egypt slaves were nearly naked.[8] Until the eighteenth century, European men and women of nobility wore ornate and layered fabrics, including intricately designed silk and lace. They donned fine hats and heels that made them similar in height, and they wore jewels, ribbons, embroidery, makeup, and wigs. In the sixteenth century, men began wearing padding to accentuate their shoulders and legs, as well as codpieces that became more exaggerated over time. While establishing gender differences in embodied presentations, snug clothing such as tights and bejeweled blouses constrained noble men's mobility, and codpieces eroticized these men's bodies by drawing attention to their genitals.[9]

Men and women's relationships to fashion in eighteenth-century America were similarly defined by class location. Both men and women of privileged classes wore powdered wigs with rings of curly hair, dressed in ornate fashions, and painted their faces. This was especially true for urbanites and courtiers, who used professional hairdressers and beautifying elixirs to create a body that "proclaimed nobility and social prestige."[10] The relationship between class, gender, and fashion in the West began to shift after the American Revolution, which ushered in new ways of thinking about the adorned body. Men and women began to eschew the costly artifices of fashion and instead put themselves forth as manly citizens and virtuous women.[11] The rejection of an aristocratic lifestyle became a democratic project that emphasized solidarity among and uniformity across classes. Psychoanalyst John Carl Flügel referred to this politically motivated throwing off of men's beauty regimes as the Great Masculine Renunciation.[12] Attempts to be beautiful were popularly criticized as reproducing inequalities among men, and a new value on work emphasized men's bodies as utilitarian. Republic ideals replaced bouffant masculinity and suggested men need not develop and display their authority because it resided inherently in them. Men's grooming, however, did not disappear altogether; rather, it went underground and was unacknowledged by a discourse of non-fashion, whereby men's appearances were considered practical rather than aesthetic.

The fashioned man reemerged in the Regency and Victorian dandies.[13] A social climber, the dandy primped and preened to signal his status as an elite man and used appearance for self-creation and the expression of individual excellence. He was a man of leisure who sought the personal feeling and public recognition of distinction through the projection of aesthetic superiority and exquisite taste. He was known for spending copious amounts of time, energy, and money on grooming his body and fashioning his garments: an impeccable three-piece linen suit, a slim tailored coat, tight cuffs, a perfectly knotted silk tie, and perhaps a tall hat and black lacquered cane.[14] While the dandy represented an air of aristocracy, the coexistence of the Romantic as an expression of individualism opened the door for men's current relationships with consumption. The value of the individual rose and became tied less to character and more to the embodied expression of identity and status. "Frequently without occupation, with no regular source of income and generally no wife or family, the dandy lived by his wits,"[15] and he signaled his manners and tastes by peacocking, or ostentatiously displaying his corporal assets. He exhibited the performative nature of self-creation, highlighting the fluidity of bodies and class displays. The Romantic, in contrast to the dandy, embodied individualism; and it is individualism that marks contemporary perceptions of consumption and fashion.

While historical analyses of the dandy focus on class, the dandy was also a racialized mode of masculinity. He represented and reinforced the social superiority of whiteness as pampered and privileged. Yet, the zoot suit—initially a black style of dress and later adapted by many Mexican Americans—was what fashion historian Colin McDowell refers to as the "first true dandy fashion of the twentieth century."[16] During World War II, black and Latino men wore sharply tailored and colorful suits, including high-wasted baggy pants that tapered at the ankles. The jackets were long and double-breasted with wide lapels and sharply padded shoulders. Zoot suits flew in the face of oppressive white middle-class norms and constraining community expectations for young men of color.[17] Similar to the peacocking dandy, zoot suiters took pride in their appearances and were known to strut down the streets for all to admire. A sign of freedom and self-determination, zoot suits were accessorized with a felt fedora or pork pie hat and feather, French-style wingtip shoes, a shiny pocket watch, and a comb.

The politicized character of the zoot suit was salient during the 1943 Zoot Suit Riots, which first erupted in Los Angeles between white sailors and young Latino men. The riots characterized racial bigotry against Latino youth, whom the press and the police described as "hoodlums" and "gangsters."[18] The riots ignited racial tensions in other parts of the country, too, with whites' attacks on Latinos spanning from San Diego to New York. Black and Latino men of the World War II-era showed how the fashioning of bodies can help disenfranchised groups to carve out distinct and self-valued racial and ethnic identities in moments of intense racism and xenophobia.

While class and race have long shaped how men relate to, dress, and groom their bodies, they were not marketed masculine identities back to them like we see today. Men purchased their suits and extoled a display of wealth or racial independence via tailored fabrics and particular grooming habits, but there were limits on men's consumption. These limitations resulted in part from the sheer lack of industrial production. That is, you can't consume what doesn't exist. Just as my father had only a few cologne options at the back of a drugstore in the 1940s, the abundance of products designed and sold specifically to men is a recent phenomenon. But also, capitalist-based consumption has been tightly tied to the cultivation of feminine aesthetics and proper womanhood; and because culturally valorized masculinity is defined in opposition to women and femininity, it has been a longer haul for corporations to convince straight men that beauty and fashion can indeed support their gender identities. A close look at manufacturers' historical attempts to create male consumers by marketing cosmetics, toiletries, and fashion to men reveals that masculinity is not something inherent to men but is a commercial identity they can purchase.

Making Way for the Man of Consumption

Early twentieth-century marketing research suggested men might purchase cosmetics if they saw them as something that enhanced rather than detracted from masculinity. Manufacturers rose to the challenge by evoking language they believed would appeal to men, such as advertising face powder as "talcum" or "aftershave." In an attempt to convince men their aftershave powder was distinctly unfeminine, a 1934 Foügere Royal advertisement depicted white men in tuxedos with slicked back hair fraternizing and sipping on brandy. The byline of the ad read: "Let's NOT join the ladies!"[19] There is scattered evidence that men dabbled in cosmetics at this time, with gay men signaling sexuality via cologne or subtle makeup,[20] wealthy bachelors using aftershave to express sophistication, and black and white working-class men appropriating fashion to parody the man about town. Yet magazines published few men's grooming product advertisements in the 1930s, and companies struggled to successfully integrate cosmetic consumption into expectations of heterosexual masculinity.[21]

Esquire magazine emerged in 1933 in the hope of producing a leisuring, consumer-oriented, middle-class masculinity.[22] As women won the right to vote and the Great Depression pushed married middle-class women into the workforce, men faced a crisis in masculinity that set the stage for manufacturers to appeal to them as consumers.[23] *Esquire* founders David Smart and William Weintraub saw men as an untapped consumer sector and set out to convince them that differentiating themselves from women did not rest in the avoidance of shopping, but rather in what they purchased and why they shopped. Evoking misogynist rhetoric of women as frivolous shoppers who over decorate and do not know what men like, *Esquire* essentialized middle-class masculinity by distinguishing men's taste from women's. Men were to stock their wet bar with drinks other than the "fluffy, multi-colored abominations" women allegedly favored, and they were to prefer a "clean, functional, machine-base design."[24] Creating sex-categorized interests that could be demonstrated through conspicuous consumption helped to dislodge shopping from femininity and set forth a map by which men could demonstrate class-appropriate, white, masculine taste and identities via their everyday purchases.

Marketers began using women's bodies in advertisements to further squelch men's fears that they may be compromising their masculinity by becoming avid and loyal consumers. By sexualizing women and positioning them next to cars, or objectifying them by showing only their legs or breasts, magazines allowed men to maintain a sense of heteromasculine superiority when flipping through advertisements for slacks or pomade. Men did not have to worry about becoming like women while consuming because they could fetishize women served up to them in the glossy pages of new men's lifestyle magazines.[25] Women became both an important corporate tool in creating a confident male consumer and a large part of men's consumer experiences. It would be another decade, though, before the social context was right to begin making grooming products a key part of men's social identities and everyday repertoires.

Men and women's relationships to cosmetics and toiletries changed with the advent of World War II. Fascism abroad seemed to threaten the American way of life, and women's beauty became synonymous with freedom and democracy at home.[26] Lipstick served as a badge of courage in times of destruction and uncertainty and a right for women who were manufacturing ammunition and flying warplanes. Cosmetics helped to draw boundaries between men and women, with state-sanctioned wartime propaganda encouraging women to maintain their femininity at a time when they were taking on new roles outside of the home. Men who enlisted in the army were expected to appear disciplined and their bodies were subject to institutional scrutiny. "Neat hair, a close shave, clean body, and polished shoes were all subject to inspection and policing."[27] To help men accomplish this on the frontlines, cosmetic corporations such as Helena Rubinstein, Inc., supplied branded toiletry kits for the U.S. Army that included "sunburn cream, camouflage makeup, and cleaner."[28] Army posts that lacked regular bathing facilities sold everything from aftershave lotion to talcum powder, lip balm, and cologne. The U.S. government promoted these products as necessary for a respectable, patriotic, gendered aesthetic; and once men returned home, toiletries became an important part of postwar masculine identities, with manufacturers using images of the white military hero to sell products to men that would make them neat and supposedly heterosexually attractive.

Men were introduced to grooming products both on and off the battlefield, and the state sanctioning of Helena Rubinstein cream and disposable Gillette razors opened the door for corporations to integrate body-disciplining products into men's everyday practices at home. After the war, however, commercial use of the soldier saw diminishing returns; and with economic shifts away from industry, the image of the new white-collar worker became a popular way to sell men toupees, gray flannel suits, no-effort exercise equipment, and novelty diets. Despite these efforts, commercial attempts to sell men cosmetic products and services were slow in coming, particularly because the beauty business was fashioned originally by and for women.

THE CREATION OF A GENDERED BEAUTY INDUSTRY AND LABOR MARKET

The beauty industry gained momentum in post-World War II America. Before this time, women concocted creams and elixirs in their homes, practicing what was known by English women in the seventeenth and eighteenth centuries as "cosmetical physics" and later as "kitchen physics."[29] Women catalogued their recipes for moisturizers and skin lighteners and shared these recipes with each other, passing them down to their daughters as part of a generalized knowledge in health remedies. White women of privilege were particularly interested in skin lighteners and powders to give the impression that, unlike laboring women, they did not tan or sweat under the harsh sun. More elaborate makeup was associated with immoral, deceitful, and promiscuous femininity, but women entrepreneurs of the late nineteenth and early twentieth century worked hard to turn this beauty culture into beauty business. Overcoming negative connotations of lipstick as for the likes of jezebels, these entrepreneurs marketed cosmetics as a form of elite feminine leisure and pleasure, and as having liberating possibilities for women. Entrepreneurial women of color often rejected Eurocentric corporal norms and framed cosmetics and grooming as a way to celebrate black beauty.[30] Some of these entrepreneurs were very successful, and their success helped to establish the market-driven beauty industry we know today and the growth of a new labor market: that of women beauty workers.

Women Entrepreneurs and the Rise of Beauty Business

Facing limited opportunities in the early twentieth-century marketplace, poor immigrant women and women of color struggled to support their families because they were ghettoized into dirty, low-paying jobs. Motivated by financial need and desperate to find ways around sexist and racist barriers to a living wage, some women turned to the informally established beauty culture to imagine new futures.[31] Women's familiarity with recipes for stirring up homemade skin moisturizers, hair elixirs, and skin lighteners provided excellent opportunities for entrepreneurship. They could manufacture and package their own products; and while many early beauty businesses failed or remained small, others gained momentum and became national operations still functioning today.

Two of the most famous early women beauty entrepreneurs were Florence Nightingale Graham and Helena Rubinstein. Graham was the daughter of English immigrants who had moved to Canada to become tenant farmers. As a young woman, she helped make ends meet by working in several low-paying jobs, including as a cashier, stenographer, and dental assistant.[32] Following her brother to New York, she landed a position as a treatment girl for a small cosmetics business and specialized in facials. At this time cosmetics were still considered taboo, especially for high-status women who did not want to be associated with promiscuity and other dubious femininities. With the proliferation of new urban pleasures such as shopping, matinees, and promenades, however, Graham saw an opportunity to integrate commercial grooming products into the bourgeois social ritual.

Graham opened a small salon in 1909 on Fifth Avenue in New York City to manufacture and sell to wealthy women an elite line of skincare products and other cosmetics. Reinventing herself under the name Elizabeth Arden, Graham practiced diction and attempted to reorganize her "habitus"—Pierre Bourdieu's concept for socially developed yet deep-seated class behaviors and tastes[33]—to evoke a refined bodily comportment and style, and ultimately to signal the elite femininity she suggested could be cultivated via the purchase and application of her products. As Elizabeth Arden, Graham served as the face of her company, projecting the image of a beautiful, well-heeled woman who was scrupulous about her appearance. Her products did not reflect women's moral death—as previous notions of cosmetics had suggested—but instead helped to signal the supposed superiority of high-status women. Graham marked herself—and by extension her products—in contrast to poor and laboring femininities, using cosmetics to create hierarchies among women.

Helena Rubinstein was Graham's biggest competitor. Coming similarly from modest beginnings, Rubinstein was Polish and opened a small storefront in Melbourne, Australia, where she sold creams she made by hand.[34] Telling her customers the creams shipped from France, she too associated her products with an elite femininity; and when she ran out of products, she would say her supplier in Europe was in the midst of manufacturing more especially for her. In this way, her customers were not simply purchasing a cream, they were purchasing a feeling of sophistication associated with the alleged French origin of her product. Rubinstein's customers slathered on the feeling of status and superiority as they applied the heavy creams she concocted and packaged in her small kitchen. Selling beauty by selling gendered class and racial privilege proved an effective strategy for redefining the meaning of women's cosmetics. Rubinstein famously declared, "There are no ugly women, only lazy ones,"[35] suggesting a moral reversal where the lack of cosmetics signaled women's slothful idleness.

For Rubinstein, selling cosmetics was about struggling against the limits of poverty and creating opportunities that did not exist for women at the time. The timing was right for Graham and Rubinstein, who took to the task of selling previously off-limit products women whipped up in the privacy of their homes. These entrepreneurs saw success in the 1920s and 1930s, when the suffragist women's movement ignited around women's attempts to expand their roles and independence. Definitions of new womanhood proliferated and, cosmetics came to symbolize the modern, self-determining woman.[36] Graham and Rubinstein therefore redefined not only their own lives but also women's needs and desires more generally; they connected women's newly emerging identities as both workers and consumers to the purchase and sale of facial creams and hair elixirs.

Women of color also turned to beauty culture in an effort to create independent work opportunities and to escape the domestic labor of white households. Madam C. J. Walker is perhaps the most well known black entrepreneur in history, and her company continues to produce cosmetics. Having worked briefly as a Poro agent selling hair and skin products for African American women, Walker opened her own company and became the first woman millionaire in the United States.[37] Black beauty business was wrapped up with racial political impulses, and Walker was hailed by civil rights activists for refusing to sell skin lighteners—recognizing the deep racist connotations of capitalizing on the fetishization of lighter skin and instead pushing for pride in black beauty.[38] Walker helped to fight for black World War I veterans and rallied together Walker agents for the Negro Silent Protest Parade.[39] She even worked alongside W.E.B. Du Bois and other black leaders and social critics to petition the government for federal antilynching legislation.

Beauty Salons and Beauty Workers

Early beauty businesswomen such as Graham, Rubinstein, and Walker were some of the largest employers of women in the United States. Both benefiting from and supporting women's struggles to redefine their roles outside of the home—whether their own home or that of their white employers'—these entrepreneurs hired women to mix and package products, and to sell products to other women. With few alternatives for reaching customers, they opened salons in which their beauty agents provided product demonstrations and educated women on the wonders of commercially produced creams and cosmetics. Walker and Rubinstein notably pioneered new systems for selling goods, including mail order, home canvassing, and pyramid organizations.[40] Women were hired for the first time to go door-to-door selling products and to recruit other women to manufacture and sell products. For the first time, women became synonymous with beauty on a commercial level as both consumers and workers. We tend to think of women as inherently predisposed to beauty products and practices, and to vanity more generally; but looking historically, it is clear that women became beauty workers as feminist politics redefined women's roles outside of the home and within the social limits on their financial agency.

Walker opened beauty salons to sell cosmetics and later staffed them with women trained to wash and style hair and to provide permanents and manicures. The growth of the hair industry during the 1920s and 1930s induced states to pass cosmetology laws regulating educational and hygienic requirements.[41] These regulations made it difficult and even illegal for women to forge a living by washing, cutting, and styling hair in their kitchens. If women wanted to meet state requirements to do hair legally, they needed to be licensed. Walker and others opened chains of beauty colleges where women learned to work with and sell hair products and to operate permanent wave machines—metal, jellyfish-looking mechanisms with wire tentacles that looked as if they belonged in a bad science fiction movie. To exude a level of professionalism, hair salons required employees to dress in crisp, white, skirted uniforms that made them similar in appearance to nurses. Keeping their hair neat at all times, these women embodied the uniformity and formality that made middle-class customers more comfortable with the hair salon while at the same time maintaining a clear status division between employee and customer.[42]

Beauty colleges promised women financial independence and glamorous jobs. In reality, however, beauticians often found themselves making little money and working in horribly dangerous and dirty conditions. Poor ventilation and exposure to toxic chemicals created health risks, particularly for black women who often labored out of stuffy basements.[43] These women suffered sore throats, headaches, and rashes. The most chronic problem, and one that continues to plague beauty workers, is foot and leg pain from standing all day and carpal tunnel syndrome from plying shears, rolling curlers, and washing hair. The cost of education associated with becoming a licensed cosmetologist weeded many women from formal beauty work, and those who stayed paid a heavy price in personal health. The conditions in which beauticians labored were sometimes so bad that even some barbers, who were threatened by the presence of hairdressers, supported organizing to improve women's working conditions and pay.

As the salon became a site for hairdressing after World War II, Graham, who had used the salon to sell her cosmetics, announced that the day of the salon was over.[44] Beauty colleges proliferated and began graduating large numbers of cosmetologists who were charged with shoring up the appearances of women according to state-sanctioned definitions of feminine patriotism. Similar to the push for women to immerse their daily identities and habits in the application of cosmetics, being well-coiffed was linked to the improvement of morale and the maintenance of civilian life on the home front. Women's investment in professional hair care rose exponentially during World War II, and the postwar economic boom meant more women had the disposable income to spend time in the salon. Complicated hairstyles of the time, including the beehive, bouffant, and poodle, were difficult to accomplish at home and made women dependent on their local hairdressers.[45] The practice of going to the hair salon became routine in both white and black women's lives; and so, a robust labor market of women beauty workers was established. These workers helped women meet cultural expectations for feminine standards of beauty and performed the emotional and psychological work of making women feel beautiful. Scholarship on beauty workers shows that women's gender, class, and racial identities are supported not only through the purchase of beauty services and application of beauty products, but also through their interactions with those women who care for and create them on the shop floor.[46]

Hair salons remained sex-segregated spaces designed for women until the late 1970s. Men frequented barbershops, which provided them a haircut in addition to a masculine environment of car magazines and homosocial banter. Yet men also have a history with the beauty industry—albeit one marked less by exploitation and more by experiences as corporate owners, salon managers, and star hairdressers. Going to great lengths to perpetuate the notion that beauty is women's business, these men reinforced the feminization of both beauty consumption and beauty work while also creating space for their own successes.

Men and the Beauty Industry

While women turned beauty into a business and remain on the frontlines of the beauty industry as service and retail workers, men are greatly responsible for the beauty industry we know today. Graham, Rubinstein, and Walker may have pulled themselves up by their bootstraps, but they are outliers. Most women who attempted to make beauty into a small empire failed. Men, on the other hand, had the social privilege, networks, and clout to propel a business into a corporation, displacing women entrepreneurs in the process. Men were more likely to be college educated and had the degrees in chemistry and business to concoct and sell cosmetics. They were also more likely than women to have the financial resources necessary to mass produce lipsticks, perfumes, and face lotions and to develop national advertising campaigns. These sorts of privileged men had the influence and social connections to convince druggists to carry their products.[47] Women who had built successful entrepreneurial beauty ventures experienced tensions with their husbands, brothers, and fathers, who often handled their companies' financial and manufacturing departments. These men were well positioned to usurp control of the beauty businesses; and when it became clear beauty could be big business, they fought women for corporate ownership. Walker's husband, for example, helped her to create advertising campaigns and to begin her mail order sale strategy—she later divorced him because he threatened her control of the company.[48] Annie Turnbo Malone established the million-dollar Poro cosmetic company, which produced products for black women, and established the Poro College for women's education in hair and beauty. Her husband and president of her company filed for divorce in 1927 and demanded that she hand ownership of her company over to him. Her company was ordered briefly into receivership by the St. Louis court. Another beauty businesswoman by the name of Harriet Hubbard Ayer divorced her husband only to have him and her daughter commit her to an asylum and then take control of her company.[49] Even

Rubinstein's beauty empire was purchased by and absorbed into Eugène Schueller's corporation, L'Oreal, after her death.[50]

Men came to own the bulk of beauty companies, but not wanting to associate themselves publicly with a feminized product, they often hired women to serve as faces of their companies and as marketing experts. These companies at times created fictitious women to give customers advice, answer inquiries, or pose as the companies' owners. One African American cosmetic company fabricated an owner, Madame Mamie Hightower, who had supposedly risen from a "mere nobody" to a "beauty culturist of international repute."[51] Women were hired as expert cultural brokers in advertising, marketing, and sales. Essentializing "the woman's viewpoint" as if it were one coherent perspective, these women offered male managers a "feminine" opinion on products and what women wanted. While early women entrepreneurs had validated beauty as a business and fashioned a willing female consumer market, men sidelined them as owners and decision makers in the beauty industry. They instead hired women in very particular and narrow ways to make themselves invisible while reaping the financial reward of cosmetic sales. Women became ghettoized as marketing informants or service workers on the shop floors of salons, spas, and, later, department stores.

Men were similarly central to the expansion of the hair industry, which, like the cosmetics industry, was built on the backs of women delegitimized as unprofessional, unskilled, and unhygienic beauty providers. During Franklin Roosevelt's New Deal, the National Recovery Administration (NRA) promoted economic resiliency through the regulation of industry pricing, production, trade practice, and labor relations.[52] Working alongside hairdressing associations, the NRA instituted sanitation codes as well as price increases and fixed hours. Created in the name of professionalism, these efforts undermined the livelihood of the numerous women kitchen beauticians and neighborhood hairdressers who charged a quarter of the cost for a home perm or traded homemade hair creams for food. New sanitation codes called for a separation of the salon from the home, where women washed customers' hair in their kitchen sinks. This compromised both women's financial resiliency and their families' abilities to meet everyday needs. Definitions of professionalism consequently delegitimized women and instead upheld white, middle-class, and masculine norms of respectability. Men "with an eye for artistry" became owners and managers of many hair salons, as well as authorities within hairdressing.[53] So, while women remained the bulk of hairdressers, men who cut hair frequently became celebrity hairdressers and were often preferred by customers. After World War II, 36,000 male veterans used the GI Bill to become hairdressers. Yet these men frequently rode the "glass escalator"[54] up to management or out of hairdressing to better paying jobs in male-dominated occupations.

Men's historical positions as owners and managers in the beauty industry tend to overshadow their more recent and growing roles as consumers. Although the 1930s saw manufacturers' failed attempts to sell men cosmetics—and male-owned beauty companies reinforced the link between beauty and women—men were an obvious untapped consumer market. In the 1950s corporations attempted to join men's identities to cosmetic consumption by replacing the image of the neat military hero with the well-coiffed corporate man. Cosmetic companies tried to convince especially middle-class white men that they would be successful at work with the right corporate look, and that this look was attainable through the purchase of pomade and other waxes and creams. Although men's fashions and cosmetic products have shifted and proliferated over the last several decades, what remains constant is the role women play as beauty providers who are responsible for the grooming and fashioning of social bodies.

MEN, MASCULINITY, AND THE CONTEMPORARY GROOMING MARKET

The Commodification of Men's Appearances

The United States saw rapid economic growth after World War II, and with it companies expanded and birthed a sizable corporate, white-collar work culture. Supplanting the previous industry-driven economy, men moved into jobs as clerks, salespeople, managers, and professionals, which by 1950 made up 37 percent of the workforce.[55] These jobs required workers to come face-to-face with customers and clients in a way factory work did not. This new organization man performed interpersonal work in the office and on the sales floor; and so, his individual capacities became secondary to appearance and personality as occupational collateral.[56] Management constantly scrutinized workers' appearances to make sure they possessed the "total package" to succeed in business. While looking "right" generally meant being white, male, tall, and "altogether average," so as to appear to be "the fellow next door," it also required having short, tidy hair, avoiding excess belly fat, and exuding physical fitness.[57] Fatness indicated a lack of character and self-control, as well as potential diminished performance, and baldness signaled a lack of success. The organization man even had a uniform: the gray flannel suit that has come to characterize white middle- and upper-middle-class masculinity of the 1950s.

Toupees, diets, and exercise equipment, such as the Relax-A-Cizor—which was supposed to sound "efficient, authoritative, and important," and like "something a real man would buy and could use"—were sold to men as necessary for cultivating a corporate appearance and to succeed in the new white-collar workplace.[58] Focusing on the maintenance and improvement of their appearances was acceptable for these men as long as it was connected to occupational ambition; and so, selling men aesthetic-enhancing fashions and cosmetics rested on the notion that men's identities revolved largely around the work they did. The idea that masculinity was tied to production and utilitarianism continued not despite of but because of men's commercial consumer habits. Manufacturers sold skin creams, strict novelty diets, and silly exercise equipment like my dad's vibrating machine as key to men's success in the workplace and distinct in purpose from women's frivolous, vanity-oriented products.

Products designed and marketed specifically for men proliferated midcentury, and men shored up their appearances in the barbershop, where they could get neat, cropped cuts to solidify their image as competent and trustworthy workers. It wasn't long before ideas about young men's aesthetics shifted, pushing them into the hair salon. In the late 1960s and 1970s, a counterculture emerged of largely middle-class white youth who eschewed the conformity of their slacked and button-upped parents.[59] At a time when civil rights and the unfair treatment of women and blacks dominated public discourse, these young people rejected their parents' conservative dress and embraced a culture of self-expression. Young white men embraced the Jesus look, with long hair and unkempt beards that signified a feminized sensitivity and rejected masculinity as strong and aggressive.[60] Men and women of color grew Afros to cast off white norms and embrace an appearance that celebrated natural black beauty. White men frequented the barbershop less as they grew their hair out. These men did not have their hair cut very often, if at all, and when they did they went to salons that staffed women, who were more familiar with cutting long hair. This hurt barbers' businesses so dramatically that some boycotted salons, especially those salons that employed longhaired men. Other barbers attempted to capitalize on this shift by recasting themselves as stylists and embracing men's changing aesthetics.

Conservatives saw this new, longhaired, white male aesthetic as a threat to masculinity, a symbol of the cultural feminization of men, and a rejection of patriotism during the Vietnam War. Veterans who came home from the war blamed antiwar, protesting hippies for their poor treatment, including the marginalization of their sacrifices abroad. Historian Lynne Luciano even found that a group of Wayne State University fraternity members gathered at a barbershop to buzz off their hair in opposition to the "emasculation of American men."[61] Long hair resulted in debates over men's sexuality, indicating that particular cultivated embodiments can challenge class and sexual boundaries in addition to taken-for-granted gender differences. The popularity of long hair for men began to fall away in the late 1970s and was followed in the 1980s by trends for white men to perm and color their hair. Following trends in the Afro, "an ironic turnout" occurred, where "permed curls were embraced by those most manly of men," including professional athletes.[62] The hair salon, which had seemed destined to remain sex segregated, saw men stream through its doors in greater numbers, helping to change the face of salons as well as who constituted beauty consumers.[63]

Hair salons produced nonthreatening masculine images to attract a robust male clientele. The tone of advertisements shifted, replacing the image of a feminine beauty salon with a more "gender neutral, business-like atmosphere," and the term "beauty" began to fall away.[64] "Beauty" is popularly associated with women's supposedly inherent and unique interests in enhancing their appearances, and so salons interested in appealing to men used "grooming" as a way to assist men in imagining themselves in these spaces (see chapter 2 for more on this). Unlike the frivolity of conspicuous "beauty" consumption, "grooming" indicates bodily care that needs to be done in order to appear clean and socially acceptable.[65] Some beauty salons therefore became "hair centers"; and as men sought out more services and a variety of hairstyles, unisex salons became popular.[66]

The 1980s saw new men's hairstyles as well as the invention of Rogaine, which drew attention to the social importance of men's hair. Drug companies originally created Rogaine as a blood pressure medication, but one side effect of the drug was hair growth. It was not too successful in helping men grow a thick bed of hair where previously there was none; nevertheless, apparently "being able to grow some hair on some men some of the time was good enough" and in 1988 men spent $200 million on hair remedies.[67] Rogaine requires daily application and has an air of feminine vanity, so advertisers sold the product using scientific and masculine language. Today, TV personality and *The Apprentice: Season One* winner, Bill Rancic, says he "took control" with Rogaine, which is "clinically proven" to help men "regrow your own hair." Hair transplants also caught on in the 1980s, with businessmen making up about 80 percent of patients at the Bosley Medical Group in Beverly Hills.[68] Manufacturers also began packaging hair dyes like "Just for Men" for male consumers who wanted to shave ten years off their appearance with a single application.

As cultural norms around men's bodies changed, so too did the treatment of the male body in commercial agendas. The 1990s solidified men's aesthetic-enhancing consumerism, with a growing array of products and professional services available to men. Hair transplants, steroids, plastic surgery, gym memberships, and libido-enhancing drugs meant men needn't feel deficient any longer.[69] The production of particularly branded clothing and cosmetic products such as hair gels and facial moisturizer also grew, and corporations used images of men's bodies to sell these things. Attempting to create bodily insecurities among men and then offer a solution, advertisements began emphasizing the male consumer of fashion and beauty, and products were tied directly to the imagined cultivation of an ideal and sometimes fetishized masculine appearance.[70] Calvin Klein's early marketing campaigns optimized this effort, showing men in tight jeans and sexy underwear, ultimately commercializing the beautiful male body.[71]

The metrosexual really took off in the early 2000s as a way for journalists to capture the growing body consciousness of class-privileged men who not only take their bodies as objects but who are brand loyal and forge masculine identities via particular clothes, beauty products, and body services. The metrosexual is similar to the dandy in his artifice, style, self-love, hedonism, and tailored sophistication more generally. The difference, however, is that the dandy is an idling man of leisure while the metrosexual is a direct descendant of both consumer identity and the muscle man of the 1980s.[72] Oscar Wilde, one of the most famous Victorian dandies, once declared, "Football is all very well a good game for rough girls, but not for delicate boys."[73]

The Growing Men's Grooming Industry

Debates over whether the meterosexual is a purely market driven representation of masculinity or actually reflects men's lived experiences and practices abound in the popular media. Some cultural commentators suggest the metrosexual has been replaced by the "retrosexual"[74] and the "übersexual," which both indicate a return to "real" masculinity. Embodied in the likes of George Clooney and Pierce Brosnan, the übersexual signifies "old-fashioned, masculine values," such as "fine wines, cigars, and red-blooded heterosexuality."[75] Comparatively, the metrosexual stands out as more feminine with an emphasis on vanity; tastes for fine wine don't really scream heterosexuality, however, and Pierce Brosnan is actually a fine oil painter and dedicated environmental activist. Aaron Traister, a writer for Salon .com, characterizes the retrosexual as embedded in consumption similar to the metrosexual, but also criticizes it as a consumption meant to "mask more traditional masculine insecurities, like being gay, or a broke loser, or a gay broke loser."[76] Sociologists Michael Messner and Jeffrey Montez de Oca discuss a sort of retrosexual image in contemporary beer and liquor advertisements; they note the ads promote the "Average Joe," "Buddy," or even a valorized version of a "Loser."[77] Despite these debates, Mark Simpson remains dedicated to the idea that the metrosexual is the way of the future for men. Gender is of course messier than all of this, with masculinities defined differently by race, class, and sexuality existing simultaneously. Not all men can afford to participate in the consumer habits that define the übersexual, for example. Each characterization of masculinity is embedded in consumerism, but they are separated by what is consumed and what this consumption signals about masculinity. While the retrosexual purchases his way into dude culture via Miller Light and Levi's Jeans, the metrosexual represents a sense of urban refinement.

Whether or not the metrosexual is an outmoded and narrowly useful term, one thing is clear: we are indeed seeing growth in both advertisements that sell designer apparel to men and products that are branded as male specific. "You can't mess with perfection, but you can moisturize it," exclaimed Shaquille O'Neil in a 2013 television commercial for Gold Bond Men's Lotion. Men are moving into salons in greater numbers to pursue a pampered experience and high-end aesthetic, and they are buying branded toiletries such as Old Spice Swagger deodorant and investing in premium "nontraditional" products, including skin creams, body moisturizers, and shower gels.[78] Market research shows that men make up a significant sector of the billion-dollar beauty industry, and companies that try to make their products irresistible to men rely on this research to understand how they can capitalize on this growing trend. Marketing data on the hair and nail industries, and on men's grooming more specifically, reveal a steady uptick in men's purchasing power in the national beauty market.

Men in the Hair Salon. From 2006 to 2014, The U.S. hair and nail industry's revenue increased over 18 percent, from $43.8 billion to $51.8 billion.[79] Market research attributes the growth of this industry to the decline of barbershops and the growing interest of well-to-do men in high-end hair care. While the recent economic recession ushered in a tightening of American purse strings, there was only a 0.4 percent dip in hair and nail salon revenue from 2008 to 2009, and men's grooming revenue grew (table 1.1). Economic trouble can actually mean big business for the beauty industry[80] with men and women pouring money into their appearances to compete in the job market and to look competent in the workplace.[81] Men and women's relationship with beauty consumption has turned a corner with more people firmly invested in the idea that their grooming experience should be a luxurious one. More than ever, they expect their hair and nail services to include "being pampered, being helped to feel good about themselves and overall satisf[ied] with the end result."[82] The willingness of people to pay premium prices for a paraffin pedicure and chic haircut is driving up revenue, to the delight of corporate executives. Not everyone is able to afford these services, however; so the growth of a luxurious grooming experience speaks to the classed meanings of high-end bodily repertoires. A haircut that includes a scalp massage and mini-facial, after all, are most easily folded into class-privileged identities and budgets.

Understanding men's forays into high-service salons or spas means taking their ever-evolving body projects seriously. These projects have helped to create new possibilities for the beauty industry just as much as they have emerged from the marketing efforts of beauty companies. As men have moved out of the barbershop,[83] there has been a bifurcation in the types of establishments to which they go for haircuts: the no-frills chain salon and the women's salon.[84] Budget chains like Supercuts pepper the landscape from the West to East Coasts and offer men quick, cheap haircuts in the smallest U.S. towns. Supercuts is popular with men, who make up 66 percent of its $1 billion per year business.[85] While technically a unisex salon, Supercuts targets men who want convenience and affordability. Great Clips, another chain store, is not well equipped to do women's hair, according to a graduate student of mine who scouted the chain salon for a potential research project. Armed with clippers and few styling products, management expects employees at Great Clips to turn clients over in mere minutes.[86]

Men who want stylish haircuts and a relaxing reprieve from the daily grind of work and family have been opting for the women's salon. Women's salons offer men a leisurely consumer experience, where they can unwind, read magazines, chat with their stylists, drink tea or wine, and get slow, methodical scalp massages. Women's salons offer clients a variety of services from haircuts and highlights to manicures and facials. While barbershops used to provide manicures,[87] well-to-do men now associate the everyday barber with working-class masculinity and do not see it as an appropriate place for them to spend time or cultivate their appearances.[88] Indeed, even with its declining numbers, the barbershop remains a staple in white working-class as well as black and Latino neighborhoods.[89]

A niche market of luxury salons is well positioned to flourish in an otherwise price competitive market where Supercuts is king. Market research states that high-service salons—whether for women, men, or both—are on the rise partly because baby boomers are resisting the signs of aging.[90] In a culture where youth is associated with vitality and aging is something to dread, men and women are opening their wallets in an effort to tighten their faces with creams and dye their greying roots. The increased demand for spa services is also linked to trends in health and wellness, and hair and nail industry reports note new opportunities for selling "value-added hair and beauty services to men."[91]

Salon owners and managers are recognizing men as important potential clients who make up an estimated one-third of consumers.[92] Even nail salons are seeing more men who want to shore up their feet for the summer sandal months and get manicures to refine their tidy professional appearances.[93] This rise in male clients is enough to begin changing the face of hair and nail salons, with salons incorporating male-specific services such as straight razor shaves and lacquer-free manicures. As especially middle- and upper-middle-class white men move away from the barbershop and seek out an array of beauty services and exceptional customer service, it is clear that men's salons such as Adonis and The Executive are well positioned to take advantage of growing trends in the beauty industry.

Even Supercuts' parent company, Regis Corporation,[94] is getting on board with the male-specific branding of beauty spaces, services, and products. Regis test-marketed a concept men's salon, RAZE, in 2010 to compete with their rival Sports Clips, a budget-friendly, sports-themed salon.[95] Although sports-loving women could foreseeably seek out and enjoy the ambience of Sports Clips, it is clear the salon caters to men in a way Supercuts does not. Sports Clips incorporates cultural markers associated with a narrow definition of masculinity, such as athletic jerseys, to provide a masculine environment and experience in addition to a cheap haircut. RAZE was supposed to appeal to men by branding the salon a space for men seeking "more." The company encouraged men to "RAZE" their "standards" and promised them "an experience, a style, a confidence." Attempting to sell sophistication on a shoestring budget, the company's website told men:

From the minute you step into RAZE until the minute you leave, you will understand why men are opting for the sophisticated and relaxing RAZE experience. With private styling stations, plush leather chairs, flat screen TVs, a beverage bar and on-trend expert advice about cuts for men, RAZE is a destination for guys who want a polished look at an affordable price. . . . Make an appointment today and experience hair cutting for today's men. All haircuts include a relaxing and complimentary shampoo, head and neck massage and hot towel treatment.[96]

Competing for a different subsector of men than Sports Clips, RAZE appeared to target men who want an all-inclusive experience: a shampoo and conditioning, haircut, neck and scalp massage, hot towel facial, and soft drink. RAZE salons have been rebranded as Roosters Men's Grooming Center, to appeal to men unsure about the salon concept, with seventy-six establishments in sixty-eight cities and twenty-one states as of September 2015.[97] The presence of a superstore in the male grooming industry points to men as a serious consumer market for companies looking to the future of beauty. Where early beauty businesses came up short in their efforts to inject beauty into men's everyday repertoires and consumer identities, recent efforts find the combination of class and gender an effective strategy for selling men not just beauty, but an experience that is luxuriously yet particularly masculine.

Men's Grooming Products. Axe. Diesel. Dove Men+Care. Nivea for Men. Beauty products for men are now household names, and young men like my brother are appearance oriented, brand conscious, and open to trying new things. Pitched as less feminine "grooming products," these brands sell sprays, creams, lotions, and gels that are not unlike women's. Exfoliate, used to slough away dead skin cells and clear up pores, is sold to men by L'Oreal's Lab Series as "scrub," and Dove Men+Care sells the combination face/body wash, "Aqua Impact." Corporate struggles to masculinize beauty have been paying off big time, with men's products taking up space on retail shelves and in some instances entire aisles. Regional grocer H-E-B, for example, created the "Man Zone" in 2009 for select stores. The Man Zone is a "male-specific beauty aisle" carrying men's cosmetics and toiletries. It is framed with "masculine blue lighting" and flanked by a TV playing sports, to apparently draw men to face wash and eye cream like moths to a flame.[98] Bloomingdale's has men's cosmetic counters that feature The Art of Shaving, L'Oreal's Lab Series, Jack Black, and Diesel, among other men's cosmetic brands. The reorganization of such retail spaces is part of corporate reshelving strategies meant to squelch men's discomfort with entering otherwise feminized spaces or with sifting through a sea of women's products to find their moisturizer or hair dye. Reshelving has proven effective for companies including Nivea, which moved their "for Men" line from skincare aisles dominated by women's products to shaving and deodorant aisles, in which men are presumably not as intimidated to venture.[99]

Companies are also renaming and repackaging products to appeal to men. Redken sells men's hair dye as "Color Camo" and Nivea packages their men's facial moisturizer, "Hydro Gel," in blue and steel gray bottles. Companies also bundle products by attaching a sample of facial moisturizer, for example, to a high-selling toiletry like deodorant. This helps introduce men to products with which they may not be familiar. Marketing researchers expect these strategies to help men's grooming product sales grow over the long term and stake its place in the larger beauty industry. In 2014, men's products saw a revenue of almost $6.3 billion, including skincare, shaving, and hair care products, as well as deodorants and bath and shower goods (table 1.1). Global beauty giant L'Oreal has invested in men and Procter & Gamble is expected to follow suit "as American males grow more comfortable with caring for their skin in a 'manly' way."[100] Much like the efforts of some early twentieth-century beauty businesses, the ways products are packaged and sold are intended to give the impression men are indeed doing something masculine by investing in the preservation and enhancement of their appearances.

Men's industry spending is rising, but this does not capture the full extent to which men are consuming beauty products. This is because, as one *Daily Mail Online* article notes, men dip into and apply their wives' and girl-friends' anti-wrinkle cream, hair styling wax, and body lotion.[101] Men are likely to identify women's products as more expensive, more luxurious, and of higher quality than their own. Borrowing women's cosmetics hints at the hidden beauty habits of men who are not yet familiar or comfortable with "for men" products. Yet men no longer have to sneak their wives' face cream. My dad dabbled in my mother's hair dye in the 1980s, but today men are shimmying up to men's cosmetic counters at Bloomingdale's or entering posh men's salons to slather on the air of class privilege and to dye their way to more youthful appearances.

One critical strategy market research fails to address, however, is the role of service workers in selling and educating men on beauty. These workers

TABLE 1.1   Men's Grooming Product Revenue, 2006–2014

Year	Revenue $USD millions
2006	4,531.7
2007	4,667.5
2008	4,771.4
2009	5,644.2
2010	5,783.3
2011	5,953.4
2012	6,031.1
2013	6,100.6
2014	6,275.3

SOURCE: Market research company, Euromonitor International (2015), estimates from official statistics, trade associations, trade press, company research, and trade interviews. Store checks and trade sources were included from 2009 to 2014.

are on the frontlines of the beauty industry and work hard to mediate men's relationships with the culturally feminized associations of beauty spaces and practices. Women have historically served as the beauty aficionados for other women, and as men become beauty industry consumers in larger numbers women remain the bulk of beauty providers, making up 94.2 percent of hairdressers, hairstylists, and cosmetologists and 85.3 percent of "miscellaneous personal appearance workers."[102] They work behind cosmetic counters, at nail stations, and in hair salons. They wax away men's unwanted body hair, shore up men's shaggy hairdos, and buff men's gnarly nails. Women who professionally groom men have emerged as a distinct occupational niche to serve a growing consumer market.

CONCLUSION

From courtiers and dandies to stylish zoot suiters and brand-obsessed metrosexuals, men have long relied on fashion and grooming to establish their social locations and relationships with others. The way men cultivate their bodies distinguish them not only from women, but also from other men along the lines of class, race, and sexuality. Embodiment thus has implications for the reproduction of social inequality, marking privileged men in distinct and visible ways. It is only recently, however, that men have had access to a plethora of beauty products and services created for and advertised specifically to them. They are marketed masculinities back to them in novel ways and there is a growing economic and cultural emphasis on cultivating a masculine appearance by purchasing the right clothes and the right cosmetic products. The rise of men's grooming as a subsector of the beauty industry allows for new exploitations and inequalities to emerge alongside men's commercial pursuit of social distinction. In this book, I investigate how Adonis and The Executive are themselves organizational efforts to reshelf beauty that deploy masculinizing efforts to lure men into the salons and to make men comfortable and confident consumers of detailed haircuts and mani-pedis.

Men's contemporary relationship to consumption and grooming is also a story about women, who first made beauty into a business and who continue to work on the frontlines of the beauty industry. Women have long sold beauty by selling classed and racialized gender, and their work helps to support commercial beauty consumption as it becomes a masculiniz-ing practice. Early efforts to sell beauty were tied largely to the cultivation of womanhood and different femininities, but we now see the prolifera-tion of corporate attempts to connect men's identities to the consumption of beauty products and services. While corporations have found it diffi-cult to sell beauty to men, the historical evolutions of men's relationships with consumption—and its meaning for developing classed and raced identities—have laid the foundation for today's grooming market. Market-ing research captures a larger cultural phenomenon, but it is how beauty gets translated and exchanged within face-to-face interactions and what these interactions mean for both the client and the worker that is the focus of this book. Men don't just buy products; associates sell them products. Men don't just get haircuts; trained and licensed stylists cut their hair. Paying attention to the workers supporting men's consumption in the beauty industry teaches us something about the way consumption and labor collide, and about how people forge identities and negotiate social relationships when new populations are folded into market activities.

2 · ROCKS GLASSES AND COLOR CAMO
Selling Beauty to Class-Privileged Men

We like to call it a modern interpretation of old-fashioned service. You'll just call it remarkable. The Executive is a grooming lounge for today's sophisticated gentleman. Whether you're looking for a close straight-razor shave, a classic cut, or even a manicure, you'll think of yourself in a whole new light after just one visit. Let us show you what it's like to be truly pampered.

—Telephone recording, The Executive

I first visited Adonis with my friend, Noah, who was having his hair highlighted to give it that sun-kissed look for the summer. It was a typical sky blue day in Southern California, and I was excited to see what exactly made Adonis a men's salon. We swung open the heavy glass front doors and slid into a couple of sleek chrome chairs trimmed with black leather. We chatted while I flipped through the magazines resting on a little round table between us: *GQ, Rolling Stone, Men's Health*. The tall, blond receptionist offered us something to drink while we waited: imported beer or a glass of wine, perhaps? I asked for water, which she brought to me in a rocks glass. I swirled the ice cubes around as if it were a glass of scotch—now all I needed was a cigar.

There was no mistaking Adonis for a women's beauty shop or even a high-service unisex salon. Clearly a lot of thought had gone into designing a space for men: modern décor, dark hardwood floors, and a Red Bull refrigerator nestled in the corner. Wood shelves lined the walls and were stocked with expensive styling products like Bumble and Bumble and the men's skin care and shaving line Jack Black. Along the right-hand wall was a bar with a beer pull and bottles of wine, and a miniature refrigerator held soda and sparkling Perrier for thirsty clients. Cheetos, pretzels, and salted peanuts were displayed in tall dispensers, and a glass case displaying an autographed basketball sat triumphantly in the middle of the room. Frosted glass separated the waiting area from the workstations so that all we could see were the snacks, the products for sale, and the pretty receptionist.

A woman in a sleeveless summer dress and with long wavy blond hair walked up to greet Noah. She smiled and gave him a tight hug as if they were old friends. I would have never guessed this was only the second time she had done his hair. He introduced her to me as Jesse, one of Adonis's senior stylists. He asked her: "Can Kristen hang out with us while I have my hair done?" Jesse nodded and invited me to follow them to her workstation, where Noah took a seat in a high-backed black chair that looked more appropriate for a space shuttle than a hair salon. A television remote was strapped to one armrest and a blow dryer was holstered on the other. I was especially impressed with the small television built into the workstation mirror. Jesse asked Noah what sort of "color camo"[1] he was looking for, and after a brief discussion she talked him into a lighter blond than he had originally wanted. She led us to the back room through a door that read, "Quiet Please, Entering Spa Area."

Jesse painted thick globs of bleach onto Noah's hair with a black silicone brush and folded the wet strands into strips of foil. Upon finishing, she positioned a state-of-the-art freestanding hair dryer over his head—the circular top rotated silently around his head, creating dry heat to quicken the hair-lightening processes. This was a far cry from the lines of hooded hair dryers stereotypically associated with women's beauty shops. Affixed to the wall in front of us were flat screen televisions connected to Xbox game systems— Noah joked that we could play a round of Grand Theft Auto. Twenty minutes later, Jesse returned to see if his hair was sufficiently blond. "Ok," she said waving us over to the shampoo bowl so that she could wash the chemicals from Noah's hair. As he hung his head back into the deep basin, he exclaimed, "Check this out!" Two small televisions playing a basketball game hung from the cabinets above him.

Adonis and The Executive emerged as the men's grooming industry began its upward swing.[2] Veronica, owner of The Executive, echoed this trend: "I took over in 2004, late 2004. . . . We sent out the right marketing message that the time is now! And we've been doing great ever since." Despite the favorable timing, Adonis and The Executive still have to compete with feminine meanings attached to beauty and bear the burden of appealing to men who are either unfamiliar with or intimidated by the idea of going to a salon. Veronica and Tyler want to convince men that they don't have to enter through a hidden back door while wearing dark sunglasses and a baseball cap; they can visit the salons confidently while maintaining— even accomplishing—structurally rewarded masculinity. But exactly how do Adonis and The Executive convince men they are patronizing what the phone recording that opens this chapter refers to as a "grooming lounge for today's sophisticated gentleman"? What are the differences between these men's salons and the conventional barbershop, the women's beauty shop, and the unisex salon? What organizational processes enable men's consumption of beauty without risking feminization? And what is it about these spaces and all the stuff in them that make these salons masculine?

The potential for gender failure is a constant threat that people are compelled to repudiate, deny, and recast.[3] The beautifying man is especially threatened by what sociologist C. J. Pascoe calls the "specter of the fag," which regulates boys' and men's behaviors so as to avoid the stigmatization of effeminacy and all that comes with it.[4] Sexuality and gender operate together to create particularly located persons, and for men who hold a great deal of status and power, their investment in beauty places at risk their privileged locations in social hierarchies. But through the process of recasting the male beauty consumer, men's bodies, identities, and social advantages become both organizational and interpersonal projects. At Adonis and The Executive, this process includes creating opportunities for men to feel masculine as they engage the people and things around them.

Adonis and The Executive are organized around a recognizable cultural symbolic order that fosters masculinizing experiences within a historically feminized institution: the salon.[5] Recoding, or regendering, the salon involves mobilizing popular notions of masculinity to make decisions about the layout and décor of the spaces and the amenities available to clients. It also involves integrating physical and linguistic markers of class privilege to support the high-status performances and social identities of a largely heterosexual, well-off, white male clientele. Serving drinks in rocks glasses, for example, symbolically references powerful performances of elite white masculinity; the availability of sports television and beer reflect nostalgic markers of straight American manhood, including things like sports bars and man caves; and video games mark Adonis specifically as a place where clients can engage in one aspect of guy culture.

Gender is created and recreated during our everyday engagement with spaces, objects, languages, and other people;[6] and so, the participatory or social character of masculinity comes into focus when looking at men's behavior at Adonis and The Executive. The salons' spaces and amenities enable clients' heteromasculinizing performances and classist projections of themselves as "sophisticated" men who sip from rocks glasses and relax in expensive leather chairs while they wait for their hair and nail appointments. These activities may or may not be dramatically at odds with their lives on a more routine basis, but in these moments, in these spaces, they take on symbolic significance.

Selling beauty to men involves acculturating them into this masculinized commercial routine. Socializing practices are built into the salon-going experience so that men learn to understand beauty, and their desire to participate in beautification practices, as class appropriate and heterosexually masculine. The work of acculturation falls on the shoulders of the frontline beauty workers who help men navigate contradictory meanings of gender; they teach men a new, feminine-free beauty language and show them how to move around the salon with confidence. These frontline workers tend to be women, whose own projections of gender become resources for mitigating men's relationships to beauty culture.

THE MEN'S SALON: A MASCULINE AND MASCULINIZING SPACE

Examining the transformation of other highly gendered places can shed light on the recoding processes of the salon. In their study of the women's gym, sociologists Maxine Leeds Craig and Rita Liberti found that "transposable gender practices may change the gender coding of an institution."

The authors are careful to avoid suggesting that a female-dominated gym is automatically a feminine organization.[7] They instead examine organizational processes and institutionalized behaviors to determine whether and in what ways the gym becomes feminized. Recoding the masculine and male-dominated gym involves instructing women on how to properly use exercise equipment and structuring the labor of employees in ways that create a nonjudgmental and noncompetitive environment for women. This environment encourages interactions between and gender identities among women that naturalize their performances and feelings of femininity.

To sell Adonis and The Executive as men's places, the owners and managers choose layouts, décors, and amenities that enable heteromasculine performances of beauty. Social theorist Michel Foucault argues that the purposeful and regulatory organization of space disciplines bodies so that people move, interact, and behave in ways that reveal the operations of power and privilege.[8] The salons' amenities allow men to engage masculinity, and by deploying classed symbols of masculinity the salons make it clear that they do not cater to all men. Adonis and The Executive eliminate working-class men without the means to afford their services and exclude men of color by focusing on scissor cuts and discouraging the use of clippers for anything besides cleaning up necklines. There are indeed gay clients at both Adonis and The Executive, but the salons are set up to appeal to and support the sexual identities of straight white men. Organizational exclusion and disciplining routines operate together to create places in which power relations—here inequality among men, as well as between men and women—are reproduced in implicit ways.

The experience of masculinity at men's salons is an embodied one, but it is clients' expressions of emotional sensations that highlight the link between physical experiences and the socio-psychological development, or internalization, of social identities. In her study of construction work, Kris Paap shows that a sensation of being (heterosexually) masculine emerges out of men's engagement in an occupation that involves strength, risk, and often times pain.[9] This makes men feel truly and naturally masculine and encourages them to consent to corporate exploitations of their bodies. Making men *feel* masculine is, for Paap, a key mechanism that helps to explain their participation in otherwise potentially harmful work. Adonis and The Executive are involved in similar diversions by producing for men the convincing feeling of being masculine while also enjoying a detailed haircut or a leisurely manicure.

The New "Old Boys' Club": A Specter of Homosociality

Several clients described The Executive as a "mini-club" for men, "a for-guys club," or an "old boys' club." The salons abound with men, clients explained, and its classed setting reminds them of private membership for-men clubs, like those at country clubs. Dan, a sixty-one-year client, told me that being surrounded by other men helped to ease his discomfort with entering The Executive. "I think the overall ambience is more comfortable because it caters to men, which removes part of the stigma." He noted that feeling he is in the "right place" comes from knowing he is in a "place for men." "The fact that it caters to men makes it more acceptable. . . . Everybody who's there is reinforcing your idea that this was a good idea." At a unisex salon, Dan explained, it is less clear men belong:

> If you go to a salon that's men and women, most of the people there are women. If you happen to go there on a day when it's just you and six women, you're thinkin', "Are these people lookin' at me and thinkin' I'm a dweeb? What's he doing here, dummy?" So I think it's just, they've made it a very comfortable place for men. . . . Why [men] choose The Executive as opposed to the women's places, or the places that cater to men and women, I think is a comfort level that they've built into the place and the fact that you look around and you get reinforced that this is a good idea. Lots of men here.

Dan's previous salon expeditions made him feel accountable to others for being a gender anomaly and as if he had failed at accomplishing masculinity. He was self-conscious about his departure from social expectations that he, as a man, should avoid symbolically feminized spaces. By emphasizing his feelings of discomfort in such salons, he reveals the socio-psychological effects of risking his masculine status and ego. This risk creates what some scholars have come to refer to as a "masculinity threat"[10] or "masculinity challenge,"[11] whereby accusations that men are feminine create distress for them and may encourage them to compensate or lash out in ways that are dangerous to both women and gay men.[12] At The Executive, Dan is surrounded by other men who are also particular about their hair, enjoy a good manicure, and want to rid their ears and noses of unsightly hair. He can relax into the space and not feel as if he has botched the social requisites of masculinity. Importantly, not just anyone surrounds Dan, but men who have similar wealth and occupational status as he does.

Alfred, another longtime client of The Executive, told me that he has his hair cut at The Executive because he enjoys sitting among well-heeled men. He likes to feel as if his tastes are similar to powerful professional men. Professional-class masculine aesthetics are tied to meticulous and detailed grooming in a way working-class masculinity is not;[13] and so, Alfred expects to see senior executives, not plumbers or taxi drivers, at The Executive: "I've been going there for years, but [what] I want to see is an older gentleman, more of a CEO or a senior executive guy who wants to look basically [how] I want to. He wants to have a nice cut. He has nice clothing. I've never seen cheap watches in the place . . . I'm a watch freak, and you look at a guy's wrist and you see a Rolex or better, an Omega or something." Alfred habitually evaluates other clients' accessories—the hardware literally adorning their bodies—to make sure they are the caliber of men he expects in the salon. He appears satisfied to project class privilege by purchasing his way into an exclusionary place that pampers men. While out of work at the time I interviewed him, he signals a professional-class status by associating with men at a "club" for the "sophisticated gentleman."

Although the men-only character of The Executive assures clients they are indeed doing masculinity appropriately—and high-status masculinity at that—they rarely interact with each other. From the moment they enter the salons, the men engage almost exclusively with women. Even as they sit facing other men while waiting for their appointments, there are newspapers and magazines to distract them from having to talk with each other. At Adonis, the chairs face the pretty receptionist and are separated by tables stacked with magazines. Clients are indeed surrounded by other men, but they don't cooperatively perform masculinity. As Dan and Alfred suggested, the presence of other well-to-do white men is important to their identities, but they do not need to fraternize with these men to feel masculine.

Adonis and The Executive become what I refer to as *specters of homosociality* not despite women's presence but because of it. On slow days there are often more women than men in the salons; and so it might seem counterintuitive to define these salons as homosocial spaces. Homosociality is key to the production of male dominance, Sharon Bird says, because it creates an environment in which men are accountable to each other for maintaining masculine norms of emotional detachment, competition, and misogyny.[14] In some contexts, though, men "interact with women in order to build and secure their ties to manliness."[15] Women become tools by which men engage in and project male power and privilege. At both Adonis and The Executive, men's beauty experiences include being waited on by women: women greet them with a smile, fetch them beer, massage their feet during the pedicure, laugh at their jokes, and compliment their haircuts to make them feel handsome. At the same time this is all part of the women's jobs, men might interpret these exchanges as sincere rather than institutionally required and structurally supported, thus creating a sort of heterosexual "temporarily yours" experience for consumer clients (see chapters 3 and 4 for more on embodied emotional work).[16]

Design, Amenities, and the Disciplining of Men's Bodies

Adonis is carefully designed to obscure men's participation in beauty. Whitney, Adonis's receptionist and manager, said that when planning the salon, Tyler "thought about a guy's mentality and what would make them feel the most comfortable." She works closely with him to develop and deliver an "elevated experience" to clients characterized by a hip environment, specialized amenities, and the feeling of being pampered. But perhaps most important in making men feel comfortable is the privacy Adonis provides them when indulging in services. Whitney continued: "We thought about . . . what would make them want to try more than just getting a haircut. That's where I think Tyler came from when designing the salon and setting up where everything was gonna be." Tyler designed the salon around men's presumed interests and insecurities; assuming that men want to purchase beauty services but do not want to be caught doing so by others, he carefully conceals the bodies of beautifying men.

Layers of privacy help Adonis to conceal men's beautification practices, and the more potentially feminizing the service, the more concealed it is (fig. 2.1). Feminizing services are difficult to fold into utilitarian discourses; while everyone needs a haircut, manicures and pedicures draw attention to corporeal vanity and pleasure. "When they get manicures and pedicures, that's a really big one the clients like because they're not sitting out in the open," Jackie, the salon's esthetician, said. "They're in the back, where people can't see them getting the manicure and pedicures, so they don't feel like they're doing something super girly." Past the mani-pedi

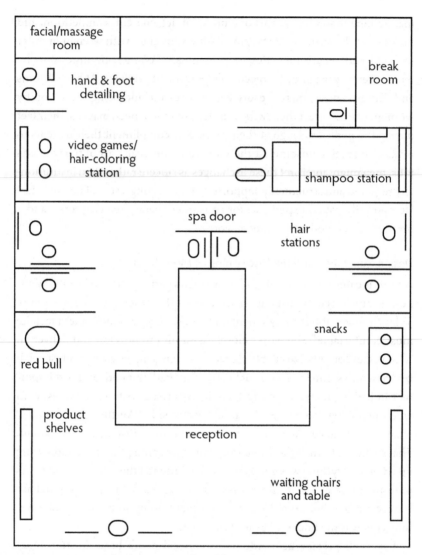

FIGURE 2.1. Layout of Adonis. Reproduced by author.

stations is a windowless room reserved for massages, waxing, and detailed facials. Waxing takes place in the back room of many women's salons, but not out of fear women will be discovered participating in feminine practices. In strip mall nail salons, women are often visible from the street through large front windows; they line the walls of these salons while technicians hunch over their hands and feet to sand off their calluses and shellac their nails. The careful layout of Adonis indicates a hierarchy of beauty practices for men in which the more feminizing services take place deep within the salon.

Noah was candid about appreciating the privacy Adonis provides him. At his previous salon, Noah's stylist made him sit outside with her while she smoked a cigarette and waited for his hair to process. He sat there publically exposed in his smock and with foils dangling from his hair. "Once in a while I'll get my hair colored, and I felt a little awkward just sitting [there]." At Adonis, however, "it's definitely more private," he said. "I like if I was to use one of the services that is not as masculine, it is private. So you wouldn't be sitting in the front window, especially on [Main Street], getting your nails done." This privacy is supposed to encourage clients to experiment with services that are new to them. An online review of one men's salon raved about the "private cutting stations": "In the back room were several other guys getting manis and pedis and sipping beer. Nice and private—a big plus." Another reviewer mentioned the importance of privacy four times in his description of a men's salon; others raved about the "private atmosphere for clients," the fact that there is "a little bit of privacy between you and the rest of the patrons," and that a manicure station "is designed with privacy in mind." One client said that the "private salon as opposed to being in a row of barber chairs makes the experience so much more relaxing and enjoyable." Privacy at men's salons also helps men like Noah to maintain the illusion that his hair is natural, as if it hasn't been colored. This hints at the performative aspect of masculinity, where to not fail at it men have to appear to not be trying.

Designed specifically as a men's salon, Adonis carefully obscures men's participation in beauty services. The Executive, on the other hand, rotated through several concepts—from a women's salon to a unisex salon—before becoming a high-end men's salon. This means Veronica has to work with the space's existing layout, which doesn't offer the same levels of privacy as Adonis. She did, however, create workstations that angled away from each other so that clients experience some separation, and the manicure station is pressed against a far back wall. Each workstation is fashioned with wood paneling, a reproduction vintage barbershop chair, and its own small television—an attempt to echo an upscale yet nostalgic masculine aesthetic. Body waxing is performed in a secluded room, but simple ear and nose waxing is done in the open. I often saw men sitting patiently with long wooden sticks protruding from their ears and noses; they read newspapers and played with their phones while waiting for the wax to harden so stylists could rip away the unwanted hair.

Popular images of women's hair salons show them chatting with each other while stylists cut and dye their hair, and reading celebrity magazines while they wait for their hair to set under hooded dryers. The salon is a place in which women socialize, develop friendships, pass the time, and catch up on gossip.[17] Historian Julie A. Willett describes barbershops similarly as organized around men's relationships. She opens her book, *Permanent Waves*, by describing her grandfather's barbershops as "all-male hangouts," where men talk to each other and casually spend the afternoon together.[18] There is a dearth of empirical work on barbershops, but the research that does exist on the subject reveals that black barbershops "play a role in the economic and physical uplift of their community" and are important places in which men extend favors to one another and socialize local youth.[19] The community-building opportunities at hair salons and barbershops inter-est researchers, with urban sociologist Ray Oldenburg referring to them as "great good places" integral to public life.[20] And except for new hipster shops,[21] the barbershop is no longer associated with the production of afflu-ence, extravagance, or a privileged, white male coiffure.[22]

The men's salons in this book echo some of the aesthetic spatial mark-ers of the corner barbershop, yet they are set up to remove the elements of community and homosocial fraternizing. At barbershops men might sit around with each other all afternoon, telling stories and offering advice (at least in popular cultural memory), and in black neighborhoods, the bar-ber might be a community leader and mentor. Barbershops, however, are dwindling in number; this appears to be especially the case in many white neighborhoods. In 2013, there were only 3,948 barbershops nationwide, while beauty salons totaled 76,203.[23] As barbershops decline and white professional men turn to the hair salon, we are losing an important place in which men have sought out conversation, friendships, and mentor-mentee relationships. Perhaps this transformation of space and relationships reflects the loosening of social ties in white, upper-middle class communities. Or perhaps these men are forging homosocial relationships in new, empirically untapped places or are increasingly relying on friendships with women to satiate their need for personal closeness. (In chapter 3, I discuss how men develop important dyadic relationships with women beauty workers who care for them emotionally and physically.)

Amenities including imported beer and *Golf* magazine act as symbolic cues to clients that Adonis and The Executive are spaces for professional well-to-do men and offer clients the opportunity to discursively and behaviorally engage heteromasculinity. New clients are delighted when receptionists offer them a Guinness beer, and one online reviewer describes a men's salon as a great place to "get faded while you get a fade." Another said the "wine, beer, or soda" make it clear his salon offers a "top-notch" experience. The word "beer" actually occurred 132 times in the 152 pages of men's salon reviews I collected. Beer helps to distinguish the salons as masculine and is not typically found in women's salons. Bonita, Adonis's sister salon located just down the road, serves its mostly female clientele coffee, tea, and sometimes champagne. Tristan Bridges uses "sexual aesthetics" to talk about men's embodied presentations,[24] but it is also an apt concept to describe manufactured objects associated with a supposed gay or straight masculine culture. Beer and drinking beer, for example, is emblematic of straight men, with television advertisements often conflating beer with heterosexual conquest and selling men on "a high holy trinity of alcohol, sports, and hegemonic masculinity."[25] The act of drinking beer aligns men, even if temporarily and imperfectly, with straight male culture while they wait for their hair appointments. And imported beer—costlier than Budweiser or Miller Light—supports men's characterizations of the salons as "classy" places that cater to their supposed superior taste and sophisticated palates.

The TVs at The Executive sit atop workstation shelves so that men can watch television while they drink their Guinness. At Adonis, the TVs are usually tuned to sports stations like ESPN, as opposed to say Bravo TV or the Oprah Winfrey Network. There are no sappy romantic movies or telenovelas on in the background. Whether or not they actually enjoy watching ESPN, sports TV provides clients an excuse for going to the salons in the first place. Dan admitted that the availability of ESPN allows him to fold his salon choice into a popularly recognizable and acceptable masculine narrative about sports. "The whole haircut experience for a lot of men is something they're uncomfortable with," he said. "And if they get to a place where they know what's goin' on and it's got kind of a cool factor, there's ball games—'This is a manly place, they got ball games!'—you know, then

I think that would keep bringing me back." When his friends ask where he gets his haircut, Dan frames his motivations as typically masculine: he goes to The Executive for the sports television and the free beer. Access to sports television helps men like Dan to obscure the fact that they are motivated by vanity. "Men are always reluctant to act like they really care," he told me. "The joke of the woman who says, 'Oh, this old thing?' when she spent forty-five minutes getting ready, men are much worse than that. Men never want to admit that they really tried to look good. The whole experience is one that they just would rather act like, 'Oh, I just go there for the ball games.'" It is significant, though, that Dan does not have his hair cut at Sports Clips, an inexpensive chain salon where the stylists dress in referee jerseys and customers watch the ballgame. This bargain chain conflates men, masculinity, and professional sports, but it does not offer the multitude of services, pampering, or stylish haircuts professional men like Dan are seeking.

Drinking beer rather than sipping tea expresses and bolsters popular beliefs about inherent gender differences and creates consumer experiences that are simultaneously classed and heterosexual. An example of what Joan Acker describes as "inequality regimes," these amenities evoke "interrelated practices, processes, actions, and meanings that result in and maintain class, gender, and racial inequalities within particular organizations."[26] The *Economist*, for instance, rests in The Executive's reception area but is a magazine not usually stocked at Supercuts, and beer is not commonly available at women's beauty salons. While ESPN might play on a small dusty television at the corner barbershop, both Adonis and The Executive offer their clients individual televisions with remote controls and a wide range of channels. Stylists told me that despite men's abilities to change the channel, they rarely do so. With sports being a heterosexual masculine institution,[27] some men might be afraid that changing the channel away from sports will signal a disinterest in football or baseball and thus will bring their sexuality under suspicion. Or perhaps some men don't change the channel because they really do enjoy watching sports. More likely, a dual process is operating where the salons are simultaneously responding to and shaping men's interests.

With the installation of Xbox game systems, a Red Bull refrigerator, and modern décor, and located beachside, Adonis reflects a stylish, contemporary guy culture. It is not a coincidence that I most often saw men who appeared to be in their late twenties and early thirties at Adonis; while

The Executive seemed to have more clients in their forties, fifties, and six-ties. Surrounded by office buildings, pricey ticky-tacky houses, and big-box stores, The Executive attracts a conservative-looking and middle-aged clientele. Conjuring up nostalgia for a time when men had more institu-tional power and men's clubs were popular places from which men ruled the world, The Executive offers professional-identified, middle-age white men an escape from the changing socio-political landscape where gender norms are shifting and critical race politics scrutinize white privilege. Here, middle- and upper-middle-class white men are at least symbolically able to maintain a sense of status by swigging imported beer, being catered to by women, and having the option to get their shoes shined by a man of color. A more identifiable masculine script, which relied on the work and recogni-tion of a wide variety of others including women and men of color, arguably existed during the period these practices and elements reference.

REDEFINING BEAUTY

Language is part of our everyday cultural symbolic order. It denotes value and relationships and thus has important implications for how we make sense of our world and who we are in it. Language and gender are mutually formed, with language establishing dichotomies that distinguish men from women and masculine from feminine. The ways we talk and are talked about are deeply gendered, reinforcing beliefs about natural differences and hier-archies between men and women[28]—as well as straight and gay, black and white—and revealing men and women's struggles with living up to cultur-ally valorized expectations of masculinity and femininity. In his book *Studs, Tools, and the Family Jewels*, Peter F. Murphy discusses the role gendered metaphors—specifically discourses of masculinity—play in our everyday lives.[29] Deploying the term "stud" establishes a man's supposed hetero-masculine identity, separates him from both women and gay men, and encourages him to participate in heterosexual aggressive behavior to prove his studliness. The routine use of such gendered language in our everyday lives supports behavior by which people create and re-create themselves in relation to others and reveals the operations of gendered power.

Selling beauty to men involves using a discourse of masculinity to mark previously feminized spaces, products, and services as "for men." Stylists at Adonis use Redken's Color Camo to dye men's hair, but they also use "color camo" to refer to men's hair dye more generally. By incorporating "color camo" into their conversations with clients, stylists communicate to men that coloring their hair can be masculine. They sell men on the exceptionality of color camo, telling clients that it is pH-balanced for men's unique chemistry. Alfred explained: "I understand from Veronica that [women's salons] don't put the right—they're used to mixing the chemicals for a woman's pH-balance of their hair, where a male is different." This is just "another thing between women and men that are [sic] different," he said.

The impulse to frame beauty as feminine naturalizes women's participation in costly, time-consuming, and sometimes painful practices at the same time it discourages men from investing in them. If men are caught beautifying, peers might stigmatize them as "sissies" or "fags," evoking defensive and exclusionary masculinity and suggesting that participating in feminized practices brings men's masculinity and heterosexuality under suspicion. Even the term "metrosexual" can be used to poke fun at a man who creams his face, obsesses over his hair, and dons fitted clothing. The revolutionary possibilities of metrosexuality are thus constrained by its association with a contemporary gender conundrum: a straight man who primps and preens.[30]

Language is a powerful normalizing mechanism that signals to men and women where their interests should lie and rewards or stigmatizes men and women differently for the same practices. The contaminating effect of beauty for straight men helps to discipline their bodies so they avoid the same products and practices in which women are applauded for investing. Adonis and The Executive therefore aim to convince men that what they are doing is unlike what women do in comparable spaces, and institutionalizing services as part of a unique "grooming" experience helps to recode "beauty" as an appropriate aspect of professional men's bodily repertoires. Class intersects with racialized gender expectations to create loopholes for professional men who see careful self-fashioning as key to both their occupational success and separation from working-class men.

"A Grooming Lounge for Today's Man"

Veronica calls The Executive a "grooming lounge" to distinguish it from women's beauty shops. This is an important detail that helps to recode her salon as a "for men" space; and she is adamant that her staff understands this as linguistically specific and reflective of genuine differences between

The Executive and women's salons. Vicky, a new hire, told me that because "Veronica calls it a 'grooming lounge,'" then, "it's not really a 'salon.'" Many employees did refer to The Executive as a "salon" during our interviews, but they were careful not to do so while interacting with clients. "Beauty" and "salon" evoke feminine associations with women in a way "grooming" does not. "Grooming" is popularly connected with men's embodied labor and conjures up images of simple corporeal maintenance rather than improvement.[31] Men even encounter the language of "grooming lounge" rather than "salon" when they are on hold during calls to The Executive.

Veronica incorporates what she calls "masculine verbiage" into the training and everyday routines of her staff. New hires undergo an eight-week educational program, during which she instructs them in the semantics of grooming, among other things. She provides stylists with a list of words to use in their interactions with clients. Vicky told me: "When I first started cutting hair there, Veronica gave us a whole paper of terminology that we have to use. She has different definitions on how to cut hair, guys' anatomy, stuff like that. . . . So instead of using women's terminology, we changed it into a more manly terminology so they understand it better." Stylists avoid asking men if they want their "bangs" trimmed and instead simply refer to "the front" of men's hair. The various sections of men's hair are "zones," drawing symbolic associations with construction sites. "Fringe" and "highlights" are completely off-limits because men have "layers," not "fringe."

Training beauty workers to act as gendered cultural mediators is key to masculinizing the beauty consumer experience for men and highlights workers' responsibilities in upholding the salons' corporate image. Similar to Arlie Hochschild's work on the corporate training of flight attendants in emotional labor,[32] Veronica expects her employees to take direction and develop a stake in the larger goals of her salon. To accomplish this, she first untrains her staff in the more typical feminine language of the hair salon—or otherwise explains it has no place at The Executive—and then encourages masculine verbiage as a routinized instrument of service to support clients' masculine identities.

Cosmetology school focuses on women, not men, stylists told me. In the classroom they learn how to do women's hair, apply women's makeup, and buff women's nails. They also learn how to talk to women during appointments, with instructors stressing the importance of personalizing interactions by asking about clients' children. Men rarely volunteer as hair models on which students can practice, and with the exception of the three licensed barbers, stylists at The Executive felt they had little previous experience doing men's hair. Veronica tells her staff they need to use a language different from what they learned in cosmetology school. "We go over male-specific terminology," she said. "We talk about how to talk to a male guest . . . 'cause we don't have women as clients. So we talk about how to take what we learn in beauty school, because we are predominantly female, and how to turn that language into male-friendly uses." The staff needs to consider men's limited experiences with beauty and abandon terminology that will surely alienate clients. When a new, less feminine expression for a product or service is difficult to identify, modifiers are attached to otherwise typical beauty terminology.

Linguistic modifiers reveal the gendered norm of words. *Male*scaping/*man*scaping and *man*lights imply that body waxing and highlighting is normally feminine and connected with women (see table 2.1). The gendered meanings of these terms help to constitute and reinforce a supposed natural contrast in men and women's interests and behaviors; as if malescaping is all that different from when women wax their body hair. Much of what it means to be a man or a woman is both directly or indirectly conveyed through language,[33] and so the salons create new terms to tackle cultural anxieties regarding the feminization of men and the breakdown of gender binaries. Since gender binaries fail to capture the complex realities and messiness of people's desires, interests, skills, opportunities, and identities—as well as their overlaps in behavior—a discourse of masculinity allows men's participation in beauty at the same time it upholds distinctions between men and

TABLE 2.1   Gendered Salon Terminology

Women's Salons	Men's Salons (Adonis/The Executive)
Salon	Grooming Lounge
Bangs	Front
Manicure	MANicure/Hand-detailing
Pedicure	Foot-detailing
Hair Coloring	Color Camo
Body Waxing	Malescaping/Manscaping
Facial	Skin detail
Highlights	Manlights

women. The symbolic power of language enables and constrains behavior by contextually associating it with appropriate displays of masculinity, such that men might hesitate to purchase a "manicure" but rave about the "hand-detailing" at The Executive.

The responsibility of routinizing a masculine verbiage of beauty falls on the salons' stylists, nail technicians, estheticians, and receptionists. One stylist at The Executive told me that men do not want "highlights" like their wives, and so she describes the coloring process to clients as a way to "cool down the gray." Adonis's use of "color camo" engenders a link between hair dye and masculinity by conjuring up images of war and corporal conquest. As Murphy notes, "For most men all relationships are tactical encounters that have to be won, lest they risk the loss of manhood."[34] The men have to "win" their encounters with beauty, otherwise their manhood might come under suspicion and damage their social privilege. At the same time men "win" at doing beauty in Adonis and The Executive, though, the constant struggle to sustain their masculinity via everyday aestheticizing reveals the vulnerable nature of masculinity.[35]

The Executive refers to the manicure as if men were caring for their cars. "At the salon, we try to—at this salon, we try to make it more male—use more masculine words, like, instead of 'manicure and pedicure,' [we say] 'hand- and feet-detailing.' Something that they would understand," said new stylist Ruth. Of course the problem is not that men do not understand what a manicure or pedicure is, but that they might associate it with women. Comparing men's bodies to machines like cars is a typical metaphor that situates them as "disembodied, efficacious piece[s] of equipment."[36] This sort of language draws from Cartesian theories on mind-body dualism to setup the disembodied man as an inverted image of the emotional, leaky, and fragile woman. Metaphors that men are machines ideologically sever them from their bodies, helping to free men from the supposed softness of bodily embellishment. Yet a machine "always runs the risk of being found defective";[37] and so, the men at Adonis and The Executive shore up their bodies to appear fully, naturally, and constantly masculine and in control of their corporeality.

The incorporation of masculine verbiage into the daily exchanges between workers and clients is supposed to help to make beauty intelligible and palatable to men. Saying that beauty jargon has to be translated for men to understand it also removes them ideologically from beauty culture and upholds the idea that men and women are so inherently different they do not even speak the same language. Teaching their employees to "talk like a guy," as Veronica puts it, reveals the social constructedness and contextual character of gender differences, such that the women demonstrate they can learn and deploy discourses of masculinity. The Executive's motto, "We talk male, understand male"[38] is meant to intercept clients' doubts about the gender of the salon and the meaning of their salon participation. Veronica said: "'[Talking] male,' everybody laughs at that, because they don't really know what that means when they read it. And it's really that my staff is trained how to speak to a man, using terms like 'linear,' keeping it masculine and referencing—like, a 'neckline' for us, we have three: 'tapered,' 'deconstructed,' and 'deemphasized.' So things like that, so men go, 'Oh, yeah, I know what that word means.' It's speaking their language."

"Linear" and "deconstructed" are mathematic and engineering descriptors, and their association with men reflects sexist ideologies and sex-segregation in both education and the workplace. The presumption that a male language even exists perpetuates stereotypes that men as a group share personality traits, interests, backgrounds, behaviors, and skills different from women,[39] and it suggests that women struggle to understand what "linear" means—and that men who struggle with it ought to have their masculinity scrutinized more closely. This vocabulary makes sense in a context where beliefs in fundamental gender differences serve both institutional and individual interests. At the same time this language might encourage men's participation in beauty, it also comes at the cost of propagating stereotypes with harmful real world consequences. We live in a world where women really do struggle for equal opportunities and recognition in STEM (Science, Technology, Engineering, Mathematics) programs and occupations.[40]

Despite this masculinizing language, beauty workers still have to reassure men they are not doing something girlie at the salons. This is especially the case for those women who provide manicures, pedicures, and body waxing. Bridget, an aesthetician and nail technician at The Executive, uses the rhetoric of "sports, women, business" to sell men manicures and pedicures. When massaging a client's hand during a manicure, she might tell them, "This is beneficial when you play golf, because you get the muscles worked and the joints of your fingers." Knowing that men who can afford a manicure or a pedicure at The Executive are likely to be professionals, she tells them that their bosses and clients will judge them by how their hands look. "I suggest to them that they have it because when they're in meetings, it's a lasting impression. 'People do notice when you've got well-groomed nails.' So I'll try and sell them on it that way, and that tends to work. If it's to do with business or women, they buy it [Laughs]." Manicures become classed gender capital by which men can navigate their workplace identities, and Bridget passes these meaning-making capabilities on to men who might find themselves justifying to others their smooth, cuticle-free hands.

Bridget uses the men's assumed investment in heterosexual conquest to reassure them of pedicures. "So I try and sell them . . . by saying that women take notice of how men's feet are. If you've got dry, cracked, ugly heels, we notice those things," she said. The pedicure becomes more than a feel good practice of vanity, leisure, and pampering; it is linked by technicians like Bridget to men's heterosexual success. These explanations provide easily accessible and socially accepted heteronormative narratives for men to manage interactions with others who notice and are critical of their tidy toes. It's hard to imagine that framing pedicures in this way would operate as heterosexual capital for working-class men. But for straight, professional white men, a pampered aesthetic is a sign of expendable income and careful aesthetic care. Men aren't "gonna turn female" if they color their hair or get a manicure, Bridget reminds them. Echoing sexist and homophobic ideas that being like a woman or a gay man is undesirable, she explained, "[It's] really a taboo. [Men] think [the] manicure and pedicure [are] female thing[s]. 'I'm not gay . . . that's for girls.'" She assures them that having one's nails done is not a gendered practice but a general necessity for men of their occupational caliber: "I'm like, 'No, you wear sandals, and you work, 'specially people that work in an office . . . they need the manicure.'"

INITIATING MEN INTO THE WORLD OF BEAUTY

The women who work at Adonis and The Executive find themselves educating men on how to move around the salons, what to expect from different services, and how to properly care for their bodies. Capitalizing on the men's interests in cultivating an appearance of affluence and distinguishing themselves as white-collar professionals, the salons attempt to make them knowledgeable and thus comfortable beauty consumers. Characterizing the salons as grooming lounges might ease men's entrée into the salons, but the work of familiarizing men with commercial beauty routines is the responsibility of workers who cultivate clients' cultural capital.

"Cultural capital" is a set of knowledge and skills developed over time through everyday experiences and group membership.[41] While it originally referred to the ability of the rich to maintain class hierarchies and to trade on their cultivated dispositions within the marketplace, this concept has been expanded to include "gender capital." Gender capital refers to those aspects of identity (e.g., knowledge, interests, resources, proclivities) within a given context that authenticate particularly gendered identities.[42] It is significant that gender capital does not work in precisely the same way for all people and in all social settings. So the kinds of gender capital that might purchase a bit of masculinity in a sports bar might be different from that demanded in the hair salon. Class and gender capital are not mutually exclusive, and so it is more accurate to say that people develop and carry with them an intersectionally informed capital. Clients at Adonis and The Executive draw from their cultivated *classed gender capital* to build the bodily repertoires and embodied appearances that establish them as properly classed men in the eyes of others, and they can draw from and trade on this capital in their everyday lives. This capital is extended as beauty workers teach them how to be proficient consumers of high-service salon services.

Salon Etiquette as Cultivated Capital

Stylists told me stories about men who had no idea how to behave in a salon. Men are unskilled in navigating the salon experience, they explained. Corey, the owner and sole stylist of a small competing men's salon, laughed as he described this experience:

> I had one guy, and he must have been, like, late thirties or forties, and I think he had been going to a Supercuts since time immemorial. When I said, "We're going to shampoo your hair," and we went to the back, he actually got on his knees and stuck his head in the bowl. He had never had his hair shampooed, so he didn't know how you're supposed to sit at the shampoo bowl. So it was like, "No, no, you've got to sit down and you lean back. It's not like washing your hair in the kitchen sink."

At Supercuts and other chain salons stylists usually wet men's hair using a plastic handheld spray bottle. This is not quite the picture of a pampered experience. While spraying men's hair might make it more manageable for stylists, it also helps them to avoid the lengthier shampoo so they can see more clients during a given shift. Kneeling in front of the shampoo bowl is probably one of Corey's more colorful examples of clueless clients, but the story highlights how men who lack salon experience may not understand the shampoo as a routine aspect of a high-service haircut. It is with repeat experiences and being educated by stylists, Corey told me, that men learn to move around the salon and to engage appropriately in beauty services.

Joshua and Ryan, who work at Adonis, and Randy, a barber at The Executive, did not discuss teaching men how to engage beauty. The women beauty providers with whom they work, however, spoke at length about walking clients through what to expect during a haircut or taught how to apply styling product. One stylist at The Executive told me that she led a first-time client to the salon's changing room—dubbed the Locker Room—so that he could stow his personal belongings and change into a smock. He indeed emerged wearing his smock . . . but nothing else. He had disrobed completely, as if he were putting on a hospital gown. She silently hoped that he had left his underwear on. Holding back her laughter—and determined to not show her shock and horror—the stylist delicately informed her client that he could keep both his pants and shirt on for the haircut. He never made the mistake again.

These women see educating men as an important part of their jobs and cast themselves as responsible for initiating clients into what one stylist called "the men concept" of commercial beauty consumption. In addition to making men more familiar with the salon experience, they also framed careful grooming as an important step in becoming a white-collar professional, so that men could develop a gendered capital compatible with their class. Corey tells his college-age clients that preparing to enter the workforce involves making sure they are "sufficiently groomed." Online reviews echo the idea that going to a full-service men's salon is "a grown-up twist on the classic boys' clubhouse" and feels like "entering the man's world of primp and pampering and . . . leaving the boyish haircut comfort zone behind." The barbershop and Supercuts comparatively become places incompatible with manhood. At Adonis, The Executive, and Corey's shop, boys become men and men become professionals.

Style, Techniques, and Products

Men are not always aware of the sorts of services available to them or why and how often they might have their hair cut or roots dyed. Beauty providers at Adonis and The Executive educate their clients on these things in hopes that the men will become self-assured clients who invest in an array of services. Many stylists find themselves teaching men the difference between a scissor cut and a clipper cut. Yet introducing men to the wonders of scissor cuts can be difficult. Corey notes: "A lot of people that come from Supercuts, they'll come in and sit down and say, 'I want a number three. I want a number four.' And they'll do that because that's the way they're trained. Supercuts trains the people to—they don't—it's for speed, so they don't really need to talk to the customer. It's like, 'What number do you want?' . . . that's what [men have] been taught." Stylists said scissors are preferable to electric clippers since they allow for a more nuanced haircut with layers and texture. Clippers restrict them to simply setting the length of the sheers—a one in the back and a three up top, perhaps—and buzzing off men's hair. They feel clippers stunt their autonomy and creativity, as well as the variety of haircuts men can purchase. This perspective ignores the creativity black barbers display when they use clippers to shave designs into men's hair and privileges their white clients' hair as ideal for styling. Clipper cuts, they say, focus less on style and experience than on price and speed.

Corey said that although some men are surprised when he pulls out a pair of shears, he assures them that scissors allow him to individualize their haircuts: "And I can do any kind of clipper cut, but I like to cut a lot with scissors, even short hair, because it gives it a more finished look, it gives it a more individualized look. It doesn't look like they just came out of a cookie cutter. And a lot of times they're surprised because I end up cutting their hair with scissors instead of buzzing it all off, which is what they're used to." After getting over their initial shock, he said, "The guys are like, 'Oh, wow! This is amazing! This is great!'" In both the interviews and online reviews, men commented on the novelty of the scissor cut. One reviewer noted that there are "No hack jobs with electric clippers . . . but all scissors." And while other reviews of men's salons note that stylists are skilled in both clippers and scissors, one particularly admires the "precision scissor cuts" and another exclaims that he "hate[s] clipper cuts." These men come to regard the more expensive scissor haircut as better to the extent that they might flinch at the sight of clippers when stylists produce them to shave the neck-line or shorten sideburns. "Sometimes I'll pick up my clippers to use them, and they'll be like, 'I don't want you to use them,'" Faith, a twenty-nine-year-old stylist at The Executive, said. A client of one men's salon wrote online that, "When I'm paying this kind of money for a haircut, I expect the stylist to actually cut my hair with scissors. Needless to say I won't be making an appointment with her again."

Teaching men that scissor cuts are preferable to clipper cuts introduces them to a supposedly superior aesthetic taste, distinguishes men's salons from typical chain stores and barbershops, and makes the salons necessary destinations for men who are invested in cultivating a professional mascu-line aesthetic. It also indicates that a white masculinity is produced within the salons, since clippers are often used to trim and style black men's hair. One stylist at Adonis even told me that since losing their one black barber the salon's already minuscule black clientele had almost disappeared. And by associating particular tools and haircuts with professionalism, stylists end up reinforcing larger cultural associations of white-collar manhood with white men. Bringing clients into the folds of the beauty industry involves racially, classed, and gender salient socializing moments. When we fail to recognize these moments, we are left with the belief that class differ-ences are somehow hardwired (such as knowledge of fine wine or prefer-ence for classical music) rather than a socially developed habitus.

Stylists also educate men in superior corporeal aesthetics by discourag-ing them from resorting to a comb-over to hide baldness. This is an issue particular to men's hair care, and stylists at Adonis and The Executive care-fully broach the subject to show men there are better ways to approach their hair—or lack thereof. Connie, a twenty-four-year-old stylist at Adonis, introduces her balding clients to the hair growth product, Kérastase, and she urges them to avoid trying to hide their baldness: "We do have Kérastase treatments at our salon that are proven to regrow hair a little bit, but not much, within six months. So sometimes we tell them about that product . . . but there's really not much they can do. We try to get people not to do the whole comb-over thing, because it just doesn't look good." Most stylists want men to know that they will look better by trimming their hair than they will by growing out long, thin strands to drape across their heads and paste into place. "I love them to death," Connie said of her clients, "But oh, my gosh, they have no hair, they're bald, and they want to grow their hair out. 'Why do you want to do that?'" She continued: "I had a couple of clients who had, like, comb-overs. One of them, I finally talked him into cutting it off, and he's happy now. But I still have clients who come in with no hair [saying], 'Yeah, I just want to grow it out.'" She said most clients take her advice, but if a client ignores her recommendation to get rid of the comb-over, then Connie will ask him to not tell others who exactly did his hair. "I have a reputation to uphold!" she exclaimed.

In addition to teaching men about scissor cuts and advising them to avoid comb-overs, stylists introduce them to an array of hair products such as waxes and sprays; and the esthetician at Adonis familiarizes them with lotions, facial washes, astringents, and exfoliates. They insist that men get overwhelmed when trying to decide which hair products are right for them and fall back on whatever products their wives use. Many clients assume that women will be discriminatory in what they purchase, and so the idea is that if it is good enough for their wives then it is good enough for them. Online articles in *The Telegraph*, the *New York Daily News*, and the *Daily Mail* discuss which women's products men should and do use, and just how much money men are costing their girlfriends by dipping into their eye cream.[43] The notion that the time is right for men to come out of the beauty closet resonates in the media, with a 2011 *Today Show* segment on "Man-fessions" covering the products "more and more men are admitting to using" and featuring a GQ editor who argues that many corporations "are marketing to women when they could be used by guys or girls."

To sell clients "for men" products, beauty workers at Adonis and The Executive tell men that the wrong product can actually cause them problems. One stylist told me: "There's a lot of people who are like, 'Oh, I just use whatever my wife gets.' One of our biggest challenges to ourselves is educating men on the difference between, 'Maybe your wife has coarse hair and she needs to use that, and you have fine hair, and that's why your hair is unruly and it doesn't do what you want it to do, because you're using the wrong thing.'" Stylists don't want to scare men away from the salon by using women's products; so they mobilize the gender essentialism underpinning the salons' brand images and commercial marketing strategies. Beauty workers at Adonis and The Executive inform men that their hair or skin is different from women's and therefore they need unique products. The popularity of biological rhetoric makes this an easily digestible and regurgitated explanation so that men can safely explore and invest in new beauty products. By informing clients that men's products are designed for the unique male body, beauty providers reinforce the notion that men and women are so biologically different that men avoid using women's hair dye lest they end up with the unclear repercussions of such a mistake. This didn't seem to be a problem for my dad, who was using my mother's hair dye in the mid-1980s. But there was also no robust male grooming industry that squirted dye into a no-fuss gray bottle and called it Color Camo.

Men's cosmetic products are packaged to conceal their likeness to women's versions of the same things. Women's "exfoliate" becomes face "scrub" for men, and gels and liquids come in containers featuring masculine imagery. Diesel cologne, for example, comes in leather-wrapped glass bottles that look like canteens: just in case men are dying of thirst in the desert? Nivea Men's Active 3 Sport Wash conjures up the image of a sweaty male athlete by featuring a runner on the bottle. Adonis carries some gender-nonspecific specialty brands, such as Bumble and Bumble, in addition to high-end men's labels like Jack Black shaving kits. The Executive sells its own line of men's products, including "grip wax" and "sports cream." Veronica commissioned these products in an effort to brand all aspects of her clients' salon experiences. The products' names make it clear what each is for: "grip wax" will keep hair in place while "sports cream" provides extra hold for the athletic man. "You can wear it while you're playing basketball," she said. Veronica explained that she wanted to label products according to "what they do," making it easy for the presumably naïve male beauty consumer to understand what they should buy as well as how and in what context they should use a particular product.

The salons sell men beauty by selling gender, and the employees end up deploying stereotypes about men to develop associations between products and a natural "maleness." Men are "gadgety," Bridget told me, and so they are interested in utilitarian things. She clarified how she uses this stereotype to peddle men's products: "I educate them on the reasons why I think they should use them, the benefits and stuff like that. They need to be told, 'You need it for this. You'll notice a difference.'" She and other employees also assure men that the salons' products are not for women. Martha, a barber at The Executive, tries to keep her descriptions of hair wax from being construed as "girlie": "I try to make it into a conversation, not a speech . . . they always think it's too girlie or sissy to find out about [products] . . . it's the same as asking for directions."

Many of the women who work at The Executive described themselves as having an important role in the larger beauty industry: they don't just clip hangnails or sell hairspray but also help to grow the men's grooming market. They initiate men into a world long familiar to women; and even though the largely female beauty staff is neither male nor white-collar, they develop identities as experts on professional-class masculine aesthetics. The stylists and nail technicians in particular ask clients to place their trust in them and to take them as knowledgeable on the requirements of a social status they are not intimately acquainted with. During her research in a Long Island beauty shop, Debra Gimlin found a similar process taking place, with both hairdressers and their professional female customers jockeying for the role of beauty expert.[44] Driven by a dedication to their social distinctions, the customers maintained class differences from their hairdressers by insisting that only they, as professionals, know how their hair should look. Similarly, women who groom men educate their clients on what it takes to cultivate a high-status, masculine embodiment and thus ultimately indoctrinate these men into the beauty industry.

The feminized character of beauty means that men are not all that motivated to express aesthetic knowledge, despite the fact that their stylists, nail technicians, and estheticians informally teach them the ins-and-outs of product chemistry and application. Men at The Executive frequently forfeited expertise to women during their interviews with me in the symbolic maintenance of gender differences. Lenny, a sixty-three-year-old fitness trainer, said women are the best at waxing away his unwanted body hair, and Finn, a thirty-two-year-old business owner, declared that "women know what they're doin' a little bit more when it comes to haircuts." Dan went so far as to characterize women beauty providers as like veterinarians because they have to decipher the hair needs of oblivious men: "You've got a patient who can't tell you what the pain is or what he doesn't like about his hair [Laughs]." The women pick up on men's deference to them as beauty proficient and expressed appreciation for clients who trust their expertise: "I just love the ones that trust me and say, 'Ok, yeah, do whatever.' It just makes it really easy. . . . They trust me," said Emily, a twenty-one-year stylist at Adonis. While the women's roles as mediators between men and beauty reinforces gender dichotomies, it also allows them to carve out identities as educators and to cultivate a sense of importance to the high-status men in their chairs.

CONCLUSION

Men risk their association with hegemonic masculine privilege at the hair salon. And although white well-to-do men have a long history with beautifying to signal racial and class status, Adonis and The Executive take on the cultural feminization of the salon to create a consumer experience that is both masculine and masculinizing. The salons have to be careful, though, because engaging the masculine threat of beauty recognizes it as much as it veils it.

By recasting the image of a feminized beautifying man—or attempting to mitigate the "specter of the fag"—both salons signal heteromasculinity with conventional symbols such as beer and sports TV. At the same time, these are not simply static symbols that rest in the mini-fridge or on the walls of the salon. They are there to be used and thus allow men's hands-on engagement with discursive notions of American guy culture. The high-end markers of masculinity, such as rocks glasses, leather seating, and *Golf* magazine go further, setting clients up to project professional-class, white heteromasculinity. Clients suggested that their engagement with a carefully gendered environment is important on a socio-psychological level because it allows them to feel appropriately masculine in the salon. This connection between *doing* and *feeling* highlights the performative and deeply sensed aspects of gender identity in these spaces.

Adonis and The Executive reject the notion that men will fail at masculinity when they have their hair "clipped and dipped," as one client put it. Both the masculine verbiage of "grooming" and the men's-only concept of the salons help to create a specter of homosociality so that clients feel they are in the right place for men like them. The repudiation of women as not belonging or even existing in these spaces provides men an accessible meaning-making rhetoric in case friends or family question their loyalty to the salons. This homosociality subordinates the women whose sex and gender become key elements of the service. It is clear that the women play important roles as cultural mediators that help men to negotiate these new spaces and to learn a new, more masculine lingo. Yet this masculinization comes at a cost: while women invest in meaningful workplace identities as educators and experts, they also end up fortifying dichotomous, hierarchical boundaries around gender, sexuality, class, and, at times, race.

3 · HETEROSEXUAL AESTHETIC LABOR

Hiring and Requiring Women Beauty Workers

Whitney was twenty-four years old and had worked as a receptionist at Adonis for three years when I met her. Recently promoted to manager, she described herself as the "organizer of everything" and emphasized the many hats she wears at the salon: "Making phone calls, greeting people," overseeing "marketing ads," and "helping the flow of communication between the front desk and the stylists and [owner]." She is responsible for upholding excellent customer service, or what she described as an "elevated experience," by "having a good phone personality" and "cater[ing] to [clients]." A large part of what Whitney does at Adonis is not written into her formal job description. In addition to scheduling appointments and welcoming clients, she also acts as the face of the salon. White, tall, and slender with light blue eyes, long blonde hair, and a penchant for plunging necklines, she is featured in the salon's commercial and on postcards enticing clients to book appointments. She stands at the reception desk on most days, visible to men waiting for appointments and to passersby who peer into the salon's large front windows from the sidewalk.

Both formal and informal labor characterize work at Adonis and The Executive. Certified cosmetologists and barbers are hired for their technical skills in wielding shears, trimming cuticles, and exfoliating skin; yet, like Whitney, they are also expected to help the salons meet branding and marketing goals. Adonis and The Executive are invested in creating and upholding high-end images that recode beauty so that it is palatable to well-to-do men and associates them with heterosexuality. Heteromasculinity relies on an accessible foil, and so the female beauty service worker becomes a resource for men's identity constructions during the haircut or manicure.

Service industry workers increasingly act as models who display the products they sell—think retail employees wearing khaki shorts at The Gap—and as decorative organizational "hardware" that adds to the overall aesthetics of a retail space.[1] In this way, service workers shape the consumer experience on the shop floor, with women in particular serving as objects of consumption by which customers engage normative gender ideologies.[2] This is often a sexualized position, with women employed at places like Adonis and The Executive suffering the demands of what I refer to as *heterosexual aesthetic labor,* whereby management draws from employees' heterosexual identities and heterogendered appearances to support both their corporate brands and their clients' social status.

Clients pick up on the salons' efforts to create a heterosexual consumer experience around men's presumed desires and fantasies. Interactions with a straight, attractive female stylist or nail technician is part of what the salons provide men, and clients exhibit entitlement to these women by flirting with and ogling them. In this way, heterosexual aesthetic labor produces and capitalizes on a straight male beauty consumer at the same time it creates dilemmas for women who do not define their occupational responsibilities, workplaces, or workplace identities as sexual. These women are expert service workers who consider themselves professionals,[3] and who hold vocational certificates from cosmetology school and barber college and possess specialized knowledge about hair follicles, "color theory" (as applied to hair coloring), and dermatological issues. Like Whitney, they invest in their formal training and skills but also find themselves navigating both the organizational demands for and interpersonal consequences of heterosexual aesthetic labor.

The women's abilities to resist sexualized definitions of their work is constrained by institutional links between heteronormative femininity and corporate success. Gender and heterosexuality intersect at the salons to produce a particular consumer experience and a particular worker, and at The Executive, class rises to the forefront of workers' expressions of heterosexual femininity to represent a beauty brand for wealthy straight clients.[4] But how exactly does heterosexual aesthetic labor organize the work of women who professionally groom men? How does this labor create challenges within worker-client interactions? And how do women navigate both the organizational and interpersonal demands made on their sexual identities and gendered appearances?

To help cultivate their brand images, corporations hire workers who already "embody the particular styles associated with their merchandise" to act as "brand representatives."[5] This hiring strategy highlights what work scholars refer to as "aesthetic labor," or corporate demands on workers' deportment, style, and speech.[6] Treating workers' bodily habitus as a commodity, corporations attempt to create the consumer at the point of interaction.[7] Customers expect to interact with employees who resemble them in terms of class, race, and gender as they peruse clothing racks at Banana Republic, for example.[8] This helps customers feel relaxed, reassuring them that they are shopping in the right place. Because high-end aesthetics are often considered white, middle-class, and conventionally gendered, aesthetic labor can result in discrimination, including the disproportionate hiring of whites and segregating employees of color out of sight in stock rooms.[9]

The role sexuality plays in shaping aesthetic labor, and thus the gendered brand and consumer experience, remains undertheorized. A few studies consider how lesbian, gay, and bisexual employees are expected to perform their sexuality at work by presenting an appearance of gender nonconformity in supposedly gay-friendly workplaces, which results in the "materialization of a visible lesbian [or gay] identity at work."[10] In her study of a lesbian bookstore, Lisa Adkins found that managers expect employees to have butch haircuts and hairy legs, and to help customers get in touch with local lesbian networks like softball leagues.[11] The identities of these service employees help to support the gender and sexual character of the bookstore and its customers.

Women beauty service workers at Adonis and The Executive suffer from corporate demands for *heterosexual* aesthetic labor, which relies on a heteronormative *gender habitus*—specifically a heterofeminine habitus. The aesthetic labor literature explains that in the retail industry, frontline service workers act as mirrors in which customers see themselves and thus come to identify with the brand and product. But men aren't supposed to identify with their female hair stylist. Rather, heterosexual aesthetic labor situates these women as available "identity resources."[12] Hiring for, developing, commodifying, and marketing heterosexual aesthetic labor situate the women salon employees as interpersonal tools by which clients can project heteromasculine identities while engaging in largely feminized consumer habits.

HIRING AND DEVELOPING A
HETEROSEXUAL GENDERED AESTHETIC

When I interviewed Trish, a twenty-nine-year-old massage therapist, she had worked at Adonis for a little over ten months. As the only lesbian, her "outsider-within"[13] status allows her a unique perspective on how heterosexual aesthetic labor drives the salon's hiring practices. She told me that it is obvious the owner, Tyler, hires only pretty straight women—with the exception of the two male stylists—and that she must have been hired by mistake. "Tyler picks girls that are attractive for sure," she said. "I don't know how I got the job. I had longer hair then, that's probably why. He didn't know I was queer then. But he definitely wants to know if they're cute . . . and if you show up without makeup on, he'll be mad." Long hair and makeup are popular indicators of heterofeminine gender identities and influence Tyler's hiring decisions, which benefit straight women who abide by normative standards of embodiment and disadvantage gender nonconformists.[14] Trish unintentionally passed for straight when she applied to Adonis, exemplifying that gender is not a fixed biological reality but rather cultivated through clothing and cosmetics. Trish sported spiky bleached blonde hair, tattoos, and a makeup-free face at the time of my research, and so she no longer met the requirements for heterosexual aesthetic labor. Freed from the demands of conventional femininity and the expectations to project a straight identity, Trish exercises aesthetic agency in a space that otherwise requires specific corporeal aesthetics. Being a message therapist also helps her opt out of this labor because unlike the stylists, she works in a small private room at the back of the salon where she isn't visible enough to threaten the salon's heterosexual image.

Tyler relies on culturally approved markers of femininity to hire the "right" sort of worker, but he also develops heterosexual aesthetic labor by policing his employees' bodies.[15] Connie, a young stylist, explained that women at Adonis have to "look good," and that Tyler sends them home to change if they don't. The women understand that looking good means appealing to the presumed heterosexual desires of their male clients. For

Mary, who also cuts hair at Adonis, this reflects the demands of the men's grooming industry more generally: "People in our industry, they're coming and guys—say they come in and there's a girl wearing just sloppy jeans with a t-shirt and tennis shoes and their hair is in a ponytail. Or you come in and the girl has her hair done, it's styled really cute, they have a lot of makeup on, they're dressed real trendy and cute, a cute little dress on or tight jeans or whatever, where would you rather go?" Other stylists echoed the idea that men choose salons based on which one provides them the most titillation. Little dresses, tight jeans, noticeable makeup, and coiffed hair, the women suggested, make Adonis a place for men who want to look at, talk to, and be touched by attractive women.

Heterosexual aesthetics look and operate differently for male workers in these places since management doesn't need or want them to appear sexually available to clients. Joshua, who was thirty-one years old and the only barber at Adonis, told me that Tyler did not regulate his appearance. "For men, I think it's different because I was the only guy for a long time, so I just made up my own [dress code]. I felt this was nice, so I'll wear this; I think it'll work, so I'll just do that. I've never been bothered. He always says, 'Oh, you always look good!'" Joshua doesn't suffer the same objectifying demands on his sexuality that the women do. Yet he still has to project a heterosexual masculine identity that does not induce clients' latent homophobic fears of being groomed by another man.[16] Ryan, a stylist and Adonis's only other male employee, and Joshua described their relationships with clients as "brotherly." At The Executive, Randy, also a barber, reportedly chats with his clients about their extramarital affairs and encourages them to brag about their heterosexual conquests while on vacation in places like Las Vegas. Heterosexual aesthetic labor at these salons thus offers clients a heteromasculine beauty experience with either a sexually available woman or a straight, friendly guy with whom to talk about women. Either way, heterosexism informs organizational labor expectations that privilege clients in the salons.

Although most of the salons' clients are indeed straight, they also have gay clients. At Adonis, women excitedly told me that gay clients often request twenty-four-year-old Ryan for their haircuts. With his California tan, blue eyes, defined muscles, and taut t-shirts, Ryan admitted: "Every once in a while I get one I feel is kind of testing the waters a little bit." He assured me, though, that flirtatious clients do not bother him "as long as they realize that's not what I'm about." His female coworkers snickered at the thought of Ryan fielding unwanted sexual attention at work, much like they do. Similar to Calvin Klein's male models that are intended to appeal to both straight and gay consumers,[17] Ryan is sometimes a dude's-dude who high-fives his straight clients and other times eye candy for gay men who want sexually appealing interactions along with their haircuts. The latter reveals the fluidity of sexuality in places defined as for one particular kind of man. Adonis is not always as straight as it appears. While branding efforts focus on heterosexual masculinity, gay clients at times occupy space where well-to-do straight men otherwise carve out privileged identities.

Heterosexual aesthetic labor less obviously influences hiring practices and work expectations at The Executive. Veronica appears more concerned than Tyler with how men's everyday entitlement to women's bodies might shape service encounters at her salon. She takes steps to mitigate this entitlement by instituting a formal dress code to create a professional aesthetic and control worker-client interactions. "Every salon has a dress code," she explained. "Ours is professional attire. No jeans. It's nothing low-cut, nothing too short, because it's a male environment. You've got to be familiar with what would provoke unwanted attention." As a result, her employees did not have stories about heterosexist hiring practices or being sent home to change into sexier outfits. This dress code, however, does not desexualize the women so much as it problematizes women's bodies over men's actions. Whether it's banning short skirts or low-cut tops, controlling women's bodies places the responsibility of diverting unwanted sexual attention from men onto women while ignoring the fact that the salon sets the stage for heterosexualized shop floor interactions.

Veronica's dress code is filtered through the salon's gendered and sexual culture so that while it is defined as purely professional on an organizational level, it becomes interpreted as heterosexually professional on the ground. Although they did not openly recognize the organizational processes that present them to clients as heterosexually available, the women do believe some men come to the salon for the "hot chicks." The women, after all, remain heterosexually appealing while upholding a classed appearance in formfitting, button-up shirts with tight black slacks or trendy off-the-shoulder tops with spandex leggings, and almost always a pair of black heels. The dress code encourages a sexualized professional aesthetic that does double-duty in a salon setup to appeal to and reinforce the distinction of straight businessmen, and thus illuminates the processes by which classed expressions of heterosexuality come to underpin the corporate image.[18] Veronica explained this link between dress code and brand: "It is discussed in our employ[ee] handbook, absolutely. We talk about attire, how you present yourself, what image is it that—the image that we have for the shop and the dress, how it goes along with that. We're a brand, and we want to support that brand in what we wear to work every day."

In addition to emphasizing a (heterofeminine) professional dress code, Veronica also creates an exclusive consumer environment by hiring college-educated women. Some stylists at Adonis were working their way through college at local public universities, but several women at The Executive already held degrees. Veronica explained that hiring college-educated women guarantees they can hold intelligent conversations with her professional-class clientele. She believes college prepares her employees to talk with clients about things like the economy, although the women said they most often chat with clients about family, sports, and popular culture. Similarly, Tyler assumes women cannot competently engage clients in small talk if they are not educated in men's interests. Assuming they are not interested in sports or current events, Tyler requests that his female employees watch CNN and ESPN at home so they are up-to-date on breaking news and the NFL draft. The role formal education plays in hiring is unclear, and women at The Executive suggested that their college degrees actually do little to enhance their conversations with clients. Yet their degrees do serve to reflect clients' educated status back to them and may very well have advantaged them over less privileged applicants when hired for the job.

COMMODIFYING AND MARKETING
WOMEN BEAUTY SERVICE WORKERS

Like Whitney, the stylists, barbers, and nail technicians at Adonis and The Executive appear on company websites and in advertising commercials, and they sometimes hit the streets to solicit new business. With the exception of the salons' websites, male employees are conspicuously absent from these marketing efforts. When the men are included, they appear as clients rather than as employees. The Executive's online gallery, for example, included a group photo of the women looking like flight attendants in matching black pencil skirts, white blouses, and orange scarves tied snuggly around their necks. Gathered on the shop floor, some women smiled at the camera while others posed as if they were cutting the hair of two men. The men sat at adjoining stations and only regular clients might recognize one as Randy and the other as Antonio, the resident shoe shiner. Making male employees invisible by disguising them as clients, such marketing efforts imply that the salon hires only attractive women and encourages existing or potential clients to imagine a grooming experience unfettered by the homophobic discomfort of being touched by another man.

A recent hire at The Executive informed me that the salon website once featured the photos and biographies of individual stylists. Mirabel, a twenty-year-old stylist wrapping-up The Executive's eight-week training program, told me that Veronica removed these photos and announced at a staff meeting that she did so to discourage clients from choosing stylists based on their looks. Veronica realized men might come to the salon partly to interact with pretty women, and so removing the photos was an effort to increase the likelihood new clients would make appointments with any stylist. The online group photo, however, helps to assure men they will certainly be booking an attractive woman when they schedule a haircut or hand detailing.

Adonis more blatantly commodifies its heterofeminine women employees. The salon's sexy online commercial attempted to lure in new clients. The commercial was so provocative that my friend, Noah, described it as "porn." It featured eight young, thin, white and Latina women—all employees at the time—clawing the front door of the salon. Music pulsed in the background and images of the women flashed by: a flicker of leg, a snarling lip as mini-skirted women slid around on stilettos trying desperately to break through the salon's glass front door. A white, well-coiffed man stood inside. His arms were crossed and he smirked confidently. A shot of Whitney licking his black polished shoe flashed across the screen before she pulled his face toward her open mouth for a passionate kiss.

This commercial looped on a small flat screen television that sat at the reception desk. I often wondered if the thumping music and erotic imagery created an uncomfortable workplace for the women, especially for Whitney who spent her days standing next to the television. The commercial made it clear that the women were not just helping to sell the salon and the salon experience to men but were themselves fetish commodities. "That's her," said one man waiting for his appointment. He looked at me while pointing excitedly at Whitney, who was either too busy to notice or pretended not to hear. He seemed thrilled to recognize the woman from the commercial; here she was in the flesh. Noah noted that the commercial is "clearly reinforcing the idea that men need to look a certain way to attract women; if you go here, you're gonna look that way, and then women are gonna be crawling all over each other to get to you." Had it featured eight women unassociated with the salon, the message would have been that Adonis's clients are irresistible to women. As it appeared, however, the commercial encouraged men to imagine sexual interactions with their own stylists and nail technicians, or with the receptionist. In November, this commercial was replaced with a slideshow of the women wearing sexy Halloween costumes at work: one wore a bee costume with a tiny tutu, knee-high black-and-yellow-striped socks, and black heels; another posed as Tom Cruise from *Risky Business*, shears in hand and sans pants, wearing only a white button-up shirt with tube socks.

The intense, pulsating commercial was not the salon's first. An earlier one had run on a local late night television channel, which Trish described as a play on commercials for porn on demand. "They had a real commercial on television. It shows a hot chick that pretty much looks like Whitney, but it wasn't Whitney, and they were like, 'Welcome to Adonis. Come on in!' It sounds like a porn hotline number at night. 'Are you bored at night? Come on in!' It sounds like that, I swear to God." Trish had seen the commercial shortly after applying to the salon, and it made her uneasy about what the owner might expect of her if she were hired.

While Trish's queer identity and embodiment allows her to escape the demands of heterosexual aesthetic labor, she still finds herself having to participate in marketing strategies that display the women as accessible sexual objects. She described an instance when Tyler required them to promote the salon during a busy summer weekend:

> Before I really started working there, there was a car show on [Main] Street, classic cars all over the place. We had to stand out in the front handing out water bottles with Adonis's label on it, trying to advertise. . . . But they all were wearing, and Tyler made me wear this, too, the tank top says "Men Wanted" on the front and it says "follow me to Adonis" on the back. I had to wear that shirt! I was gonna shoot myself. I was like, "There's no way!" And you're walking around and the guys were like, "Men *wanted*?"

This marketing strategy invited men to approach the women as if they were personally soliciting sexual attention. While she was surely not the only woman who felt uncomfortable, Trish found it especially difficult being heterosexual bait to attract a straight male clientele. As a new hire, though, she did not want to upset her boss, and so she complied—although she removed the tank top as soon as she could.

THE INTERACTIVE CONSEQUENCES OF HETEROSEXUAL AESTHETIC LABOR

Men who pursue stylish haircuts and soft hands in the commercial beauty industry seem to challenge the specter of the fag,[19] which encourages boys and men to exercise heterosexuality lest they become sissies. Heterosexuality, after all, is a key characteristic of hegemonic masculinity, which enjoys a spot at the top of the gender totem pole. Men who behave in ways that meet expectations of hegemonic masculinity are, at least momentarily, marked as real men. These behaviors include displays of toughness and competition in work, sports, and the aggressive or otherwise entitled sexual pursuit of women. Few men actually live up to these expectations, which are exemplified in the images of James Bond and Don Draper. But the closer men come to the "charmed circle" of sexuality,[20] the more they reap the rewards of gender privilege. Men who do hegemonic masculinity access respect, honor, and "successful claim[s] to authority."[21] Performances of heteromasculinity include men making sexually suggestive comments to or about women, invading women's personal space, bragging to other men about their heterosexual exploits, and slinging homophobic remarks.[22] At Adonis and The Executive, men's association with hegemonic masculinity is created during their exchanges with women beauty workers.

Women Beauty Workers as Sexually Available

"What could be done to improve my experience? Maybe if the women were topless!" Paul, a middle-aged client of The Executive, answered one of my survey questions aloud. He looked at me and grinned, adding, "Just kidding." I felt embarrassed for the women working within earshot, and I noticed that nobody admonished him for making such an inappropriate comment. But why would they? The women are in the business of making men feel comfortable in the salon. Randy wasn't there that day, and even if he was, I doubt he would pipe up. Challenging Paul would mean challenging his identity as a masculine sexual subject, and the last thing management wants is for men to not feel masculine. The salon's carefully cultivated consumer experience does not include reprimands for sexist remarks. In a space designed to cater to men's presumed heterosexual desires, such remarks are neither out of context nor out of the ordinary.

I skimmed through Paul's survey after he left the salon. Surprisingly, none of his answers reflected the remark about topless stylists. In fact, only three of the sixty-nine men who filled out my survey at The Executive wrote anything that might be considered sexual. One man noted that he goes to The Executive for the "hot girls," while a second explained that he likes his stylist to be "good-looking" in addition to being a good conversationalist who is skilled with scissors. A third responded to the question about what would improve his salon experience: "Nothing that is legal!" followed by a winky-face. Perhaps the survey's formality or the employees' presence discouraged candor. Either way, it is clear the stylists' organizationally prescribed sexual availability is not lost on the men. One client compared women stylists to attractive waitresses: "You might think this place is like eating at some restaurant where you go because of the waitresses, but this place has substance!" In other words, while women who cut men's hair in high-service salons are skilled, their looks help to get men through the doors.

Clients use the women to frame their salon visits as heterosexually motivated and to pitch the salons to other men. Online reviewers tell their friends that men's salons have "hot girls" in addition to providing stylish haircuts, men's magazines, and flat screen televisions. Finn, a thirty-two-year-old client of The Executive, noted that men emphasize their heterosexuality to avoid coming under suspicion of being gay. "If you tell your friends where you get your hair cut . . . they assume it's a little bit sideways or maybe you lean *that* way." Highlighting women's presence eases men's homophobic insecurities, reassuring both themselves and others of their heterosexuality. One online reviewer explained that men's salons are "basically the same as Supercuts. That is if you substitute the portly elderly woman for attractive women, and substitute the waiting room's crappy fashion magazines for a beer, snacks, video games, and substitute the barely serviceable haircut for a great haircut." In other words, men's salons like Adonis and The Executive are nothing like Supercuts, neither in terms of gender nor class. This depiction of Supercuts as a place lacking amenities and where old, over-weight women deliver clients poor haircuts reinforces stereotypes of chain salons as inadequate places for the pursuit of style, overlooks variations in clients' experiences at these places, and couches men's salon experience in terms of women's heterosexual appeal. Classed gender differences at Super-cuts are represented instead as sexual differences,[23] whereby sexy young women signify a high-end aesthetic and thus mark men's salon as places for middle- and upper-middle-class straight guys.

Online reviews also characterize high-service men's salons as classy places for men who care about how they look. A review of one salon exclaims, "If you are male and you care about your hair, this is it!" At first glance, this dichotomy between men who "care" and men who presumably don't care gives the impression that choosing a luxury salon is based entirely on indi-vidual taste. Dividing men along these lines, however, ignores the social origins of taste and the fact that not all men can afford a $39 haircut. Finn explains that for some men in some places, the investment in commer-cial salon services is accepted and commonplace rather than an affront to masculinity. "I'm from a small town [where] people would probably be like, 'You guys—you're goin' *where* to get your hair cut?' I think down in our area now, I don't think it's a thing. You're a married guy and you're in business and you get a sharp haircut in the business center." The sexual ori-entation of men who go to salons is open to suspicion in Finn's hometown. For married men working in business and living in an urban area, though, patronizing places like Adonis or The Executive make sense. Paying for styl-ish haircuts that cost two or three times more than those at Supercuts reflect self-care, a "business" aesthetic, and moral superiority, and help to reproduce class inequalities by separating privileged men from working-class men.[24]

Entitlement to Women's Bodies and Labor

Amit, a graduate student at a local university, was surprised to have a male stylist during his first visit to Leather, a competing men's salon in South-ern California. Leather was decorated in cool metals and light woods, and it was known locally to serve the father of an international pop star. "I thought they only had women," he exclaimed, "and they seem to advertise it as being attractive young women, but my guy was a *guy*!" A self-identified feminist, Amit explained that he does not want an arousing heterosexual interaction at the salon and is comfortable with a male stylist. Being touched by another man doesn't intimidate him, he insisted, but he was surprised to see a man working in a homosocial environment branded as heteromasculine.

Clients at Adonis and The Executive similarly expected women to work in men's salons. To them a men's salon is obviously a place for heterosexual interactions. This logic conflates the purchase of body-oriented service work with sex and gender with sexuality. Much like in bars and nightclubs, the salon clients seem to think acting heterosexually aggressive and demonstrating entitlement to women's bodies make them authentically male and appropriately masculine. Conversely, *not* ogling, touching, or otherwise flirting with women might be experienced by men as moments of gender failure. When I asked men at The Executive what they like about the salon, many of them pointed to the attractive women. Fifty-one-year-old Calvin said of his experience, "This may sound a little piggish. It is—frankly, the fact that all the women in there are really attractive adds to it." I had expected the men to appear uncomfortable talking to me about their delight in having attractive stylists and manicurists. But since gender is a performance accomplished publicly—so that others witness it—not shirking from expressing heterosexual attraction made it clear I was not to think they were gay. Some men did clarify that they would leave the salon if they were not also receiving excellent customer service, superior haircuts, and the luxuriousness of hot towel treatments and scalp massages.

While some men framed the attractive female staff as an "added benefit" of going to Adonis or The Executive, others treated women as the main attraction. Here's what Dan, who likes that the salon is a "place for men," had to say:

> Now, I should say, though, Monique is a stunning blonde. And I have a couple of friends who also go to Monique, or went to Monique, and I know that [her appearance] mattered to them. I mean, one of 'em said, "I walked in and I didn't have an appointment, and I saw her and I said, 'What's her name?' and they told me, and I said, 'When does she have an appointment?'" [Laughs] They said "Not until three o'clock." He said, "Fine, I'll be back at three o'clock." I said "Really?" This guy is fifty years old. Monique was twenty-four, twenty-five. And he says, "Yeah, it's just—she's just fun to look at."

Like a "kid in a candy store" (as Noah describes the experience for men), this client unabashedly chose his stylist from the shop floor for her appearance.

He wanted to look at her while he had his hair cut, and he did not hesitate to order her up at the reception desk, even arranging his schedule around her availability.

At Adonis and The Executive, men purchase interactions with heterosexually attractive women obliged to smile and serve them beer in addition to expertly style their hair. "In order to keep clients, you treat them like a king," Mary, at Adonis, said. "You are like their servant. 'What can I get you to drink?'" Evoking the discourse of "service as servitude,"[25] she suggested clients purchase not only women's technical skills in hair or nails, but also unequal gender relations that subordinate women who fetch them beer and keep the television tuned to ESPN. Warren, a thirty-four-year-old self-proclaimed "Mr. Mom," agreed, "There's a tremendous amount of sex appeal at The Executive, and most guys, that's what they like. They like being waited on hand and foot by beautiful women." Warren makes it clear that it is difficult, if not impossible, to distinguish clients' desires for sexy straight female stylists from feelings of dominance. The men, he suggested, want to be waited on by agreeable women, even if these women are occupationally required and organizationally encouraged to wait on them. In this way, feeling masculine—or the socio-psychological consequences of gender—is tied to in-the-flesh interactions that are for sale at the salons.

Exceptions: Older Women, Lesbian Women

Despite racial and ethnic differences, the work experiences of women employed at Adonis and The Executive are shaped by the organizational demands and interpersonal consequences of heterosexual aesthetic labor. Yet two women I interviewed escaped these demands. Martha, the sixty-year-old barber at The Executive, is aware that her age affects who her customers are: "And for me, being older, it's gonna take a man—I have a lot of younger clients . . . but the younger [women] have more older ones. [Laughs] I don't have a lot of older guys." In a culture where a woman's heterosexual value diminishes with age, Martha recognized she does not operate under the same informal labor demands as her younger coworkers. While they serve men's heterosexual desires and imaginations, she is a mother figure who listens and gives advice to her clients. "I think that a lot of the older gentlemen feel better and more peppier around the younger girls," she explained, "and I think a lot of the guys see me as a mom. They just like it. A lot of them say, 'You're like a cool mom.'" While heterosexuality is not integral to her labor, gender still structures Martha's work within the salon. Acting at times as the resident mother hen, she nurtures her clients and coworkers and shares with them her life lessons. Finn sees Martha every few weeks for a haircut and likes that she is "older than me and has kids that are my age and she'll—like, I like talking to people that have a lot of wisdom." Her age also allows him to avoid backlash from his wife. "Then when your wife says, 'Who cut your hair?' 'A nice, sixty-year-old woman.' You don't have to say she's a cute twenty-five-year-old girl. . . . You have nothin' to feel bad about."

I mentioned earlier that Trish, the lesbian massage therapist at Adonis, also escapes the demands of heterosexual aesthetic labor. She described how men waiting for their appointments ogle Whitney, who works the front desk, and explains that she does not have to deal with such behavior: "My world is totally different." Tyler does not require Trish to wear heterosexually appealing clothing. "I mean, I'm in scrubs for Christ's sake," she said. While she wears scrubs as her massage therapist uniform, this had not always been the case. "I used to just wear jeans and a t-shirt." Wearing her one-size-fits-all unisex scrubs helps to relieve Trish of the expectation to sexually appeal to clients and allows her some comfort at work, making her situation similar to that of the male stylists. In fact, she said that she will not stand for Tyler telling her otherwise: "There's not a push to wear scrubs at all, and there's not a push away from scrubs, either. If he did, I would not be there."

Martha and Trish revealed that not all women hired to groom men experience organizational or interpersonal demands on their sexuality. Being older and lesbian allows them the freedom to carve out alternative, less objectifying relationships with their clients. These outliers indicate the salons can and do make room for other embodied femininities and sexual identities. This does not mean that Martha and Trish are better able to emphasize their technical skills over informal gendered labor demands. Martha related to many of her young male clients as a surrogate mother, and Trish often found herself acting as a sounding board for the men's status-enhancing comments. Bragging about their expensive possessions, the men project classed displays of masculinity while Trish massages their shoulders. "They have a lot of things they want to be proud of, because they're, like, a wealthier type. . . . I had a client the other day that not necessarily bragged but pretty much told me the things he owns and, like, how pretty much successful he's been, how he has this fancy car." She also finds herself navigating men's emotional releases while giving them massages. "The guys will come in with issues that maybe they don't want to talk to their girlfriends about or their wives. Like, I'm their therapist, mentally and physically. . . . I've had people, like, cry in there, where it's really obvious, like, 'OK,' you have to tell them everything's gonna be fine. It's like a motherly type [of care]." While these women do not have to negotiate the interpersonal effects of heterosexual aesthetic labor, their work is still largely gendered as they, along with the other women workers, find themselves performing emotional labor that is both reassuring and ego-enhancing for the men (see chapter 4). In this way, their roles as accommodating and nurturing women allow clients to maintain entitlement to gendered labor without the expression of heterosexual desire.

NEGOTIATING THE EFFECTS OF HETEROSEXUAL AESTHETIC LABOR

Men's salons sell more than just haircuts and hairspray. They sell the time and skill of beauty service workers who hold licenses to clip cuticles, trim bangs, exfoliate skin, and wax away unwanted hair. In cosmetology school, they learned how to sterilize equipment and design haircuts to flatter particular face shapes, and in barber college some became legally qualified to give straight-razor shaves. While many salons charge clients more to have their hair cut by a master stylist, and celebrity stylists hold social prestige (such as Peter Lamas, who cut Jackie Onassis's hair), the women who work at Adonis and The Executive struggle daily to contain the delegitimizing effects of heterosexual aesthetic labor and to uphold their professional identities.

Beauty providers' formal education and specialized knowledge situate them as expert service workers who are more skilled and better paid than waiters and retail associates. Yet they are not included in the professional knowledge economy occupied by most of their clients, who are judges, accountants, civil engineers, and software developers. Women already have more difficulties than men acquiring professional recognition because others see them as women first, rather than as skilled workers.[26] The shop floor presents "a minefield of threats to the dignity and virtue of female workers";[27] and while beauty workers often find themselves navigating unequal race and class relationships with female clients,[28] women who groom men end up rejecting their sexual objectification to maintain legitimacy and dignity. The degree to which they can sharply define these boundaries with the men, however, is constrained by the fact that the salons' commerce, as well as the workers' own financial success, depends on maintaining uninterrupted interactions and ongoing relationships with clients.

Service workers at times reimagine, redefine, and remake humiliating and subordinating work experiences in ways that give them a sense of dignity and power, and that allows them to maintain professional identities.[29] This is particularly tricky in workplaces that require employees to touch clients' bodies, and for whom work might be linked to sexual labor.[30] Friends and family often probe the women about what it is like to work on men, and so, by the time I asked them to describe their experiences, they were well practiced in answering questions about their relationships with the men in their chairs. Clear patterns emerged in their descriptions of heterosexualized encounters with clients, including the evocation of professionalizing rhetoric and emotional labor to deal with the situations, and of essentialism to frame men as sexual animals. These strategies allow the women to save face by justifying and naturalizing the role heterosexual aesthetic labor plays in worker-client interactions.

Professionalizing Rhetoric and Emotional Labor

While women working at both salons refer to themselves as professionals, and to their respective salons as professional places, The Executive's female stylists used this rhetoric most often. This reflects Veronica's preoccupation with her clients' occupational status and the overall appearance of her salon. At staff meetings, on the salon's webpage, and in her everyday interactions with stylists, she discusses just how important professionalism is to the salon's brand image. She invites her stylists to cast their everyday interactions with clients as "professional," providing them the rhetoric they need to reframe the objectifying and exploitive effects of heterosexual aesthetic labor. Despite the many ways in which their male clients sexualize them, many women insist their clients see them as fellow professionals or evoke emotional labor to maintain seamless interactions with clients

When I asked June, a stylist, if clients ever flirt with her, she said, "For the most part, they know they're in a professional business, so they're not gonna cross the line." June gives clients credit for knowing the difference between appropriate and inappropriate behavior and denies that they cross the line. She paints a picture of a respectful clientele that does not see the women as sexualized "geishas," "girl-next-door-hotties," or "eye candy,"— which is how some online reviewers describe women working at men's salons. She instead suggested that men self-regulate their behavior because they respect the salon as a professional place. Thirty-five-year-old stylist Kendra hinted that sexuality can enter the stylist-client interaction, but only in limited ways. "It's not that big of a deal. We're in a professional environment, so it's not gonna get out of hand." Both June and Kendra suggested that the classed aesthetics of the salon has a professionalizing effect on the stylist-client interaction.[31] The salon's clean lines, dark wood, and leather are after all reminiscent of a business office. These workers assume the men act professionally (meaning not sexual) in their own workplaces, and so they will behave similarly at the salon. Imagining that clients see them and the salons as professional allow women working at both Adonis and The Executive to represent their work as devoid of "excessive merger" or over-rapport,[32] thus casting the stylist-client relationship as rooted in understood though unspoken intimacy boundaries.[33]

Claiming that men don't bring sexuality into the salon fails to reflect the fact that sexuality organizes corporations, that men regularly objectify women in the workplace, and that displays of heterosexuality are a common resource for men to solidify their association with hegemonic masculinity. Men have a history of bringing sexuality into the workplace by objectifying the women they work with.[34] These displays of heterosexuality as sexual entitlement to women's bodies reflect their privileged place in the gender order.[35] And research shows that employees informally agree upon an acceptable degree of sexuality at work, depending on who is evoking sexuality and how.[36] Employees understand sexuality as sexual harassment when evoked by people in positions of power within an organization. Minority men might also find themselves labeled as harassers in an environment where women define similar behavior by white men as unproblematic.[37] But what does it mean when customers or clients sexualize their interactions with service workers, especially when those workers compromise their sense of professionalism if they allow such behavior yet risk valuable income if they resist it?

Cracks in the stylists' depictions of clients as sexually constrained appear when they have to remind men that they are professionals and would appreciate if the men would treat them as such. As soon as she assures me that men "are not gonna cross the line," June admits that she sometimes has to remind clients that she is serious about her work. "I think you just have to be really up front with it. [I tell them,] 'I take my job seriously. This is a professional place. I would appreciate if you just leave it at that,'" she said. While June demonstrates a limited amount of authority in this example, the degree to which a stylist can enforce intimacy boundaries at work is constrained by the fact that they must maintain seamless, ongoing relationships with clients to be successful. The women more often than not find themselves "coyly deflecting" men's remarks with laughter.[38] "I'll jokingly say, if they get a little loud, I tease them, I'm like, 'This isn't that type of place,'" Kendra told me.

From the receptionists and stylists to the massage therapist and nail technicians, women involved in professional men's grooming participate in emotional labor, whereby they suppress their disgust and frustration with clients to make the men feel good. Emotions, Arlie Hochschild shows us, are work.[39] Corporations require and commodify employees' emotions to provide good customer service and thus to create a loyal clientele. We can see this in the smiles of flight attendants as they interact with rude and demanding customers,[40] and in the deference of Korean nail technicians who cater to well-to-do white women.[41] Salons are spaces in which clients come to both feel good and trim their shaggy manes, and so women working at Adonis and The Executive are required to provide men an easygoing consumer experience that excludes chastising them for unwelcome sexual behavior. Bridget, at The Executive, described one client who came in every few weeks to have his back waxed. He was a "real creeper," she said, and he made her uncomfortable with the "stuff he comes out with": "Yeah, me and my girlfriend go at it all night, so it gets a bit hot with all that back hair." Overhearing Bridget's story, Kendra said with disgust, "Gosh, you get, like, the worst clients ever!" Bridget was uncomfortable with her client's remarks, but she ignored them to create an enjoyable salon experience for him. "So yeah, after hearing something like that, it's like, I don't want to hear that. I still have to do my job, but my heart's not in it. That can be difficult sometimes because I still have to do my job and pretend I'm liking it, but I'm not really enjoying it." Workers' silence is important in meeting clients' expectations of good service. This silence requires workers to be subordinate to the men, who freely make sexual remarks and account sexual tales. This culture of silence is epitomized in a small sign hanging above the shampoo bowls at Adonis: "This is your clients [sic] time to relax . . . do not engage in conversation." The customer is always right in service work, and so selling products and services means providing clients privileged consumer experiences, especially in high-end retail.

Emotional labor helps workers to manage not only their clients' feelings but also the feelings of jealous wives and girlfriends who are suspicious of their partners' relationships with the women at the salon. One day while Brinn, a stylish receptionist at The Executive, was making her usual string of confirmation calls, I overheard her assurances that she was calling from a legitimate salon:

> Brinn hangs up the phone and sighs, "You know what really bothers me? When I make a confirmation call and the guys' wife says, 'This is Joe's *wife*.' I'm not here to steal your man, lady!" She tells me that this happens quite often because wives and girlfriends do not know their husbands or boyfriends are expecting a confirmation call from the salon and wonder who the woman calling is. "Yeah, they're like, 'Who *is* this?!' And I tell them I am calling from The Executive about their hair appointment."

Wives and girlfriends often question the legitimacy of Brinn's relationship with clients. To defend herself, she frames these suspicions as irrational and overlooks the institutionalized character of heterosexuality in the salon.

Isabel, who had worked at The Executive for three years, told me that she constantly reminds clients' wives that although she touches and talks with their husbands, she is a professional within a professional space. She assures the women that they have nothing to be worried about and put one wife at ease by saying, "'Oh, my God, now I know you, he knows you, that is so neat!' I'm like, 'Now you know where your husband comes is a really, really respect[able] salon, it's really professional, it's nothing to be scared [of].'" Slippages between bodily grooming and sex work create insecure wives who sometimes force the stylists to explain the nature of their interactions with their husbands. They hold the women beauty providers accountable for participating in heterosocial work that involves intimate (although one-way) exchanges of touch and talk. Because the male barbers and stylists are not organizationally sexualized and commodified, they do not have to manage these jealousies. In fact, Joshua, at Adonis, said that he forms close friendships with his clients and their wives. On more than one occasion, a client has invited him to join his family for a weekend barbeque. He believes that by virtue of being a man, he can build these sorts of relationships with clients. His female colleagues, he said, are denied respect from clients because their relationships with the men always come under suspicion. Clients' wives and girlfriends seem to ask: What are the women's motivations for working in men's grooming? Whereas Joshua noted, "There's no contingency upon [my relationship with clients]. It's not where, 'My hair stylist is this cute girl,' or whatever."

In addition to evoking professionalizing rhetoric and emotional labor to mitigate clients' sexual remarks and wives' suspicions, the women deploy two professionalizing protocols:[42] monitoring what they wear to work and drawing social boundaries between themselves and their clients. Jesse, who colored Noah's hair during my first trip to Adonis, explained that stylists should avoid wearing revealing clothing. "You wouldn't want to wear anything that's too crazy, too short or whatever, be uncomfortable all day working around all men." This implies that women should expect catcalls, flirting, ogling, and other sexually aggressive behavior from men, and that this behavior is both normal and natural. Not only does this idea relieve men of responsibility for their actions, but it also limits women's ability to label unwanted sexual attention as harassment.[43] Instead of understanding clients' sexual remarks as a reflection of men's dominant position in the salons and in the gender hierarchy more generally, women scrutinize their own attire as well as that of their female coworkers.

Elsie, a stylist at Adonis, told me that it is the women's individual responsibility to avoid unwanted comments. They should be careful not to give off "that vibe," she said, which makes "guys react in that way." Evoking a victim blaming discourse, Elsie and other women personalize their experiences of unwanted sexual behavior rather than evoking a critical attitude toward how exactly the salons' management, culture, and marketing messages encourage heteronormative performances at the salon. Their ability to protect themselves from unwanted sexual attention by monitoring what they wear is limited by larger institutionalized demands for a heterosexual corporeal aesthetic and identity. The women are left to personally control men's structurally and organizationally supported heterosexual entitlement and dominating behavior.

The social boundaries stylists draw between themselves and clients to maintain their professionalism includes creating informal rules such as not dating clients. Mary said that she sometimes socializes with her clients in large groups. However, she has a strict "no dating" rule by which she regulates her relationships with the men. "I try to keep it professional in certain ways . . . now that I'm single, I have been asked out a few times, and that is just—it's really tempting. Some of them are really good-looking and have a lot going for them, and it would be great. But for me, I just don't think I could date a client. So I kind of keep it on that level." Many women refuse to fraternize with their clients in any way outside the salon. Bridget, for example, told me, "I don't really have any clients I have friendships with, no. I like to keep my work life separate from my private life. That's why I've said I'll never date a client." These boundaries help to separate the women's personal and work lives, and to ultimately maintain a sense of professionalism.

Essentializing Men's Bad Behavior

Stylists deploy essentializing rhetoric to make a non-issue of men's heteromasculine performances. Essentialism is a view by which people explain things as having "real" and "true" attributes, and it is popularly used to discuss gender in ways that reduce men and women, and masculinity and femininity, to static biological predispositions. Jesse, referred to by coworkers as the resident "MILF,"[44] said that the "guys" she works on are mostly "harmless." "Maybe some guys might [flirt] . . . but they might just be like that. I'd say 90 percent of the time they're probably married anyway. I don't think—they're pretty harmless, I would say . . . not too many creepers . . . not really anymore." Framing men's flirting as natural because they "might just be like that" implies they should be expected to act this way. Jesse also suggested that a client's married status protects him from being a "creeper" and gives him a pass to make "harmless" sexual remarks. Race and class, however, affect the way people label unwanted sexual behavior,[45] so that while a married status might protect white, financially privileged men from negative labels, it is less likely that a stylist would frame poor or minority men's advances as "harmless." The same racist and classist stereotypes that cast poor men and men of color as criminal, dangerous, and hypersexual also allow white men's subordinating behavior. Veteran stylists most often engaged in this essentializing rhetoric, indicating that they have moved through a period of adjustment in which they became accustomed to the salons' sexual culture.[46] For example, while stylists told me that men flirt with them, ask them on dates, send them flowers, and ogle at their breasts, it was largely stylists who had worked in men's grooming for a few years that said these things happened in the past and rarely, if ever, still occur.

Not all stylists cast men's sexual behavior as harmless, though. New hires at The Executive expressed surprise and frustration with the sexualizing behavior management and clients expected them to put up with and reciprocate. Two new stylists mentioned that Veronica encourages them to greet clients with a hug. Nell, a stylist who had been in training at The Executive for two months when I met her, said, "Veronica does encourage that we hug our clients. I have a big problem with that. But that's only because I feel that's outside my job duties, in a sense." Ruth, another newcomer, also explained that in an occupation where workers are expected to touch their clients, it is important to know how to keep an interaction from becoming sexual. "Because touching, being in this industry, you have to be comfortable with touching people. But everybody knows if it's a weird touch or not, or where it crosses the line into being unprofessional." Managerial encouragement for stylists to hug their clients shows the women's jobs as beauty workers involve more than cutting hair, it includes serving up a gendered and heterosexualized consumer experience.

As women become accustomed to a certain degree of sexuality within their interactions with clients, they begin framing men's sexual remarks in terms of biological inclinations or leave the salon for another job. The idea that men are slaves to their libidos resonates in popular rhetoric and is easily adopted by stylists to make sense of why men sexualize their encounters, and it helps to explain why the women fail to resist this sexualization. Emily told me that men are "wired" to sexually objectify women, but that she and the other stylists at Adonis try not to encourage this. "Obviously, a lot of guys probably come in here because there are all these—'Hot chicks' gonna cut my hair, it's gonna be so cool,'" she said. "Like, we don't act like, 'Oooh!' Like a Playboy Bunny. . . . So, I'm sure they have it in their heads, guys are wired like that, but we don't play into it." Despite having clients who treat her as a sexually available "Playboy Bunny," Emily maintains a sense of professionalism by avoiding over-rapport with her clients and coyly minimizes the effects of their behavior. She said, "I have this one guy and [during the head massage] he's like, 'unnnh, unnnh.' And I'm like, 'OK, I get it, you like the head massage. You don't have to make those groaning noises, please.'"

Since a mini-facial accompanies the haircut at Adonis, Emily worked within the limitations of a job that privileges clients' feelings, muffling his moans by placing a warm washcloth over his face.

Aggie, a stylist at The Executive, insisted that men's objectifying reflex is so deeply ingrained that they may not even realize they are staring at women or "subconsciously" think doing so is OK. Aggie's stories about clients who make objectifying remarks reveal how organizationally supported heterosexuality shapes men's interactions with stylists, as well as how stylists use essentialist ideas about sex-linked biological urges to excuse this behavior.

KRISTEN: So, do you feel like some of them are there because you're an attractive woman and—

AGGIE: Not me personally, but just, you know, not, like, maybe subconsciously. Some of them subconsciously [Laughs]. They'll be like, "Can I have an appointment with the blonde with the big boobs? I don't remember her name." It's like, "Oh, so you remember that, but you don't remember her name?!" But that's guys.

KRISTEN: Has anybody said that?

AGGIE: Oh, yeah. The receptionists get that probably more than—we never hear that, because they would never—well, most of them wouldn't say that to us, but, yeah, sure. You see them—if they're following somebody—if you're watching them follow—as we lead them to the Locker Room or whatever, you'll see them, like doing the look.

KRISTEN: The check-out look?

AGGIE: Sometimes. But that's guys. It's one lesson. It's just they're—it's guys.

Reduced to their body parts by male clients, women attempt to neutralize or minimize blatant objectification by saying it's a matter of "men being men." Individuals, the popular media, and the courtroom have all relied on the idea that men have uncontrollable heterosexual urges to excuse sexual harassment, rape, and the general degradation of women by men. Essentialism places the burden of sexual harassment on women—who must brush off harmful remarks and make sense of harmful behavior—rather than making men accountable for their actions. Setting men's behavior up as "natural" reinforces the larger gender order in which men exercise power over women's bodies and workplaces create heterosexual cultures.

Stylists evoke the "caveman mystique" to help essentialize men's hetero-sexual aggressions.[47] This is the idea that men are so close to their primitive roots that they cannot control their sex drives and are inherently promiscuous skirt chasers. Men's misogynistic behavior is cast as natural rather than as a consequence of larger structures that allow and encourage them to define women in terms of their heterofeminine appeal. Sociologists understand that the performance of hegemonic masculinity via displays of heterosexuality comes at the expense of women's subjectivity, where women are denied full personhood and their value is determined by their sexual relationship to men. At the same time, by explaining away men's bad behavior, women are able to maintain financially beneficial, although personally and professionally problematic, interactions with their clients.

Holly, a young stylist and nail technician at Adonis, catches men staring at her breasts while she stands in front of them to cut their bangs. "Whatever," she says. "[I] laugh it off. They're fricking guys. Like my boyfriend says, boys think with their unh-unh. They don't think with their brains most of the time. So I just try to keep that in mind, and I'm like, whatever." Laughter is a form of emotional labor that helps women to manage uncomfortable or unwanted sexual attention from men.[48] But at the same time laughter reveals women's discomfort, it may also be a symptom of women's socialized submissiveness. Holly asserts that because these men are her bread and butter, putting up with their staring is financially beneficial. "If they want to come back to me, hey, I'm makin' money off 'em." The bulk of beauty workers' salaries consist of commissions and tips, and so they literally cannot afford to resist men's sexual behavior, and frame their silence as capitalizing on men's heterosexuality. Using the caveman mystique to mark men as a lower form unable to think with their brains also allows women a sense of superiority to men who hold most of the cards.

Drawing the Line

When clients "cross the line," women end up redirecting the flow of power, redefining the situation, and challenging men's entitlement to their identities and bodies. Sociologists tend to focus on the horrible, the atrocities experienced by the most marginalized people. Barbara Risman argues that while sociologists importantly investigate how inequality is reproduced, it is just as important to explore under what circumstances change takes place.[49] Unveiling the mechanisms of change reveals how organizational policies may be revised to promote more egalitarian relationships between workers and their clients, as well as between workers and management. Under what conditions do women problematize men's behavior? When do they challenge larger taken-for-granted gender relations that situate men as entitled subjects and women as sexually available?

Cutting and styling hair, buffing nails, giving massages, and waxing away men's unwanted hair take place largely in private dyadic interactions. Women define men's sexualizing behavior as problematic when it moves beyond these dyadic interactions. By making public romantic advances, men highlight the heterosexual nature of the women's work and threaten to humiliate and delegitimize them as experts. Jackie, Adonis's esthetician who provides facials, told me stories about clients sending her flowers, wine, and other gifts, and Gabrielle, a stylist at Adonis, said men sometimes spend an exorbitant amount of time at the salon or make back-to-back appointments. These instances, while rare, motivate stylists to "draw the line" by reporting these men to management or by explicitly and directly setting the limits of intimacy. These moments of resistance reveal the circumstances under which women evoke agency and break through the structures that keep them silent, docile, and sexually available, even though doing so places these women at risk of losing clients.

Gabrielle told me that clients "just want to look at you," and that this inflates the men's egos. A lot of men flirt with her, she said, but, "when they talk to me and I feel uncomfortable, I automatically tell the front desk, 'This is the last time I've done a haircut [with this client]. I don't want to see him on my books ever.' We write it and [it] comes out of the computer, and then you don't get that client." Gabrielle gave me the impression that she is indeed in charge of her interactions with clients, yet she had reported only two clients during her two and a half years at Adonis. This is because the client has to go beyond the usual flirting, ogling, or crude sexual remark to be defined by stylists as a problem. She went on to say that a client who crosses the line is not actually refused service but simply passed on to another stylist. One client would not leave her chair for nearly two hours after she had finished his haircut. He continued to extend his cut, asking her to take a bit more off here and there. It was evident to her that he just wanted to flirt. Gabrielle tried to end the encounter by telling the client she would have to charge him for three separate haircuts. When that didn't work, she suggested that perhaps she was not the best stylist for him, and that someone else might more effectively "satisfy your needs." The next day, she came into work to find that he had scheduled yet another appointment with her for the following day. Frustrated, she complained to Tyler, "When he called the next day, and I told my boss he made an appointment with me again for the next day, I'm like, 'I'm not gonna cut his hair. I don't want to have anything to do with him.' . . . So, my boss said to [the male stylists], 'You guys are the escort guys. If he comes in you escort him [out].'"

Although Gabrielle indeed no longer had to deal with this client, Tyler did not refuse him service or speak with him about his inappropriate behavior. He merely redirected the problem to the male stylists. Being a bouncer is not part of these men's job descriptions, and it places them in a potentially risky situation in which they have to confront an aggressive client. Positioning male beauty workers as bouncers conflates sex and gender by assuming the men are comfortable with physical force and that they are and should be protectors of women. Troublesome clients are dealt with individually despite the fact such problems are created and perpetuated on an organizational level. When men publically evoke organizationally sanctioned heteromasculine entitlement, they bring the women's informal labor requirements into stark relief. Reporting problem clients to management is an unusual practice at Adonis or The Executive, but doing so highlights the limits on what women will put up with from clients and to what extent they will uphold the salons' heterosexual brand image and consumer experience.

Jackie told me that she confronts problem clients directly, calling them at home to inform them of her boundaries.

JACKIE: Recently one of the clients has sent me flowers. He came in and he had left his phone number, so I called and I was like, "Hey, I do want you to know, I told you before, I have a boyfriend. I just want you to understand that it's not like that. I don't want you to get the wrong idea. You're more than welcome to come back any time. This doesn't change anything, but I just want you to know that it's a work friendship. I am your esthetician and that's it. Anything more than that, it just can't happen." But it can be uncomfortable, to an extent, kind of like, "Dang, I don't want to see this person!"

KRISTEN: Is it tough to make that phone call?

JACKIE: Yes. It's either, you write a note or make a phone call. Just to make it easy, you make the phone call. You have to draw the line, you really do.

Coyly deflecting a client's unwanted attention or reiterating one's professionalism aims to diffuse an uncomfortable situation while also maintaining a jovial relationship. "Drawing the line," however, risks embarrassing and alienating clients. Jackie told her client that she hopes he will feel free to come back any time, although she confessed to me that she does not want to see him again. If he does come back she will have to undertake emotional labor to show that he is indeed welcome and manage any backlash that might come from her rejecting his advances and reeducating him on her professionalism and subjectivity. She can only hope that her call will either drive him away altogether or make clear her unwillingness to conform to the informal organizational requirements to seem available—her attempt to create a less sexualized and objectified relationship with the client.

CONCLUSION

Service employees negotiate sexuality at work, and at Adonis and The Executive this means navigating and reimagining the demands of heterosexual aesthetic labor. Possessing and projecting a heterofeminine habitus informally shapes women's suitability and work in these places, but it is also bolstered by more formal rules around women's appearances and how they should treat clients. Women's informal labor is crucial to forging a brand image that redefines the beauty consumer experience as masculinizing, and heterosexuality shapes this labor to create women workers who are fetishized commodities and men workers who are like brothers. While not all clients flirt with their nail technicians or have extramarital affairs about which to brag to their barbers and stylists, these sorts of behaviors are salient in consumer spaces where masculinity is built into the brand.

Cracks in women's meaning-making rhetoric reveal the constraining effects of corporate branding efforts and the extent to which women can exercise agency at work. While they generally imagine a heterosexualized professionalism, their agency is particularly elastic when clients' sexual behavior moves beyond the private worker-client interaction. In these instances, they refuse to become a heterosexual character, or "other woman," in these men's lives. The other woman status, however, has just as much to do with emotional and physical labor as it does with women acting as heterosexual identity resources.

4 · HAIR CARE

Emotional Labor and Touching Rules in Men's Grooming

Petite with long dark hair, Isabel walked out from her workstation. She wore slim black slacks with a button-up shirt and bracelets dangled from her wrists. Her heels clicked loudly on the cement floor as she made her way toward a tall, white, middle-aged man with salt-and-pepper hair who stood at reception. She was the only Mexican stylist working at The Executive, and her accent was heavy as she greeted her client. "Hi, Dean!" she exclaimed with a wide grin, "How are you?" Isabel wrapped her arms around his shoulders, pulling him toward her for a hug. He smiled back, "Hi, Isabel," and kissed her on the cheek. She asked how his wife was and chastised him playfully for not seeing her sooner, "It's been *too* long." Waving him toward the shop floor, Isabel invited him to "Come on back." She placed her hand between his shoulder blades and led him to the Locker Room so he could change into a smock.

After changing and slipping on a pair of complimentary black sandals, Dean met Isabel at the shampoo bowl. She kicked back his chair. Dean laid his head into the deep basin, closed his eyes, and moaned softly as Isabel shampooed and conditioned his hair. She ran warm water over his head and dug her nails gently into his scalp. Isabel's shampoos are the envy of Vicky, a twenty-six-year-old stylist in training. "Isabel is very touchy-feely. She gets in there and does the job," she told me. Some of Isabel's clients are so relaxed during the shampoo that they fall asleep in the bowl—a point of pride for her.

During the haircut, Isabel asked Dean about his family and his upcoming vacation, and, as a financial advisor, he gave her pointers on managing her investments during the economic recession. She laughed at his jokes and ruffled her fingers through his hair to see how the newly trimmed layers fell. When she was finished cutting his hair, Isabel shampooed Dean once more so that he could go back to work without fine bits of hair flaking onto his white shirt. She rubbed styling product around in her palms and quickly but skillfully molded his hair into a neat part. He evaluated his cut, and Isabel assured him that it made his eyes "pop." Dean agreed that he liked his new cut before heading back to the Locker Room to change out of his smock and back into his dress shoes. He paid for his haircut at reception, where Isabel told him, "It was nice to see you again, Dean!" She asked if he needed any product and reminded him to pre-book his next appointment. He assured her he would. They hugged once more before parting.[1]

Isabel's familiar and intimate interactions with her clients appear effortless, and Vicky described her as "touchy-feely," as if it were part of Isabel's natural predisposition. Caring for clients, though, is corporately promoted as a key component of her job and a tertiary commodity included in the men's salon experience. Adonis and The Executive are service-oriented corporations focused on selling haircuts, manicures, facials, and body waxing. Mousse, styling wax, shaving cream, and other cosmetics are secondary products, although clients at times stop by the salons just to purchase these items. Caring, while not classified by the salons as a commodity that men can choose from a menu—and which does not have a price tag—is built into each service. The feeling of being cared for both emotionally and physically is just as much for sale at these men's salons as a haircut.

"Care. Verb. Care is a Verb," Veronica, owner of The Executive told me. "It's an active process to cut hair and genuinely care. I mean, you can care about somebody, right, 'It's great to see you,' but unless your actions and your words look the same . . . if that care didn't come through . . . you could give a great haircut, but if they didn't feel it, they're not going to come back." Veronica encourages her employees to deliberately and authentically care for clients. And it is the women employed at Adonis and The Executive who especially understand their jobs as providing more than a good haircut; they provide men a leisurely beauty experience characterized by care.[2] But what exactly does it mean to care? How does a corporate emphasis on masculinizing beauty impact the organization, experience, and meaning of this care work? How do the beauty providers at these salons create caring interactions and relationships with the men in their chairs? Does everyone care equally?

As industrial production in the United States has given way to a new service economy, caring has become a fundamental aspect of face-to-face work.[3] Flight attendants do not just walk passengers through the safety regulations of commercial flights or serve peanuts and Coke; they also greet passengers, express deference ("yes, sir" or "yes, ma'am"), and apologize for bumpy flights.[4] Restaurant waitstaff members do not just take orders, fill drinks, and run food; they also ask customers how their days have been, remember regulars' orders, and sometimes slip customers free desserts.[5] Similarly, Roxy, a barber at The Executive, described her job as providing clients "more than just a haircut." "You wear a lot of hats when you're cutting hair here," she said. "You're basically in charge of making them feel really good when they leave."

But unlike flight attendants and restaurant waitstaff members, beauty providers develop ongoing relationships with many clients, where they see them every few weeks and provide them with luxurious, pampered consumer experiences that involve high degrees of talk and touch.[6] Previous beauty work research explores how hairdressers conduct "emotional labor," managing their own feelings to make customers happy and to navigate unequal relationships with clients,[7] but it overlooks the importance of physical contact and how systems of gender and sexuality differently shape labor when men, instead of women, are beauty consumers and beauty providers.

With the exception of Miliann Kang's work in Korean nail salons,[8] sociologists have been slow to develop theoretical frameworks for understanding how emotions and bodies come together in service work. She shows that the sorts of nail salons in which technicians work (white or black; high-service or working class) determines how they speak to and touch clients. At Adonis and The Executive, who is doing the touching affects the ways beauty providers labor. Men who work as barbers and stylists in these salons, for example, often avoid massaging their clients' scalp during the shampoo. While Kang shows that bodily and emotional exchanges operate simultaneously in beauty work, I am interested in how and under what conditions emotional labor becomes a function of touch. That is, "feeling rules," which script workers' emotional labor,[9] and *touching rules* operate dialectically to shape what service work looks like and what it means.

The production of care at Adonis and The Executive offers clients a holistic pampered experience involving both emotional and physical caressing, and stylists act as "hairapists" who listen to clients' personal problems at the same time they trim men's beards and bangs.[10] This pampering meets the class expectations of well-to-do men and involves caring, attentive, and obsequious labor in high-service organizations governed by white, middle-class feeling rules. Pampering is tied to raced and classed expectations of deference, and thus to the reproduction of group hierarchies,[11] but it is also a term and a process associated with feminized corporeality. On the one hand, the women beauty providers at Adonis and The Executive were clear that the salons offer men a place to be "pampered like women," and that they have to manage the tensions of simultaneously providing a class appropriate and heteromasculine experience. Pampering in the men's grooming industry includes men's consumption of what I describe as *heterofeminine care work*, the institutionalization of (often hidden) caring strategies, and women's deployment of masculinizing emotional labor to mitigate the pillorying effects of physical pampering. Men employed at Adonis and The Executive, on the other hand, risk the potentially feminizing association of beauty with their clients, and so their interactions with the men in their chairs are shaped by feeling rules and touching rules that shore up their own masculinities as well as that of their clients. As Veronica noted previously, workers' "actions" and "words" need to look the same to produce a cared-for experience that is appropriately masculinized, heterosexualized, and classed for the client and the worker.

THE GENDER OF CARE WORK

Women are considered to be naturally nurturing, and with that comes images of a bosomy mother figure who is compelled to care for others. Studies of care at work, however, show that care is built into or required by occupations often filled by women who are hired for their supposed inherent sympathy and gentleness. We might find ourselves believing women make the best primary school teachers because they are purportedly predisposed to be more patient and supportive than men. Men, in contrast, are generally considered to make good administrators (e.g., principals, deans, chancellors) because they are thought to be more decisive and better leaders than women. Such narrow assumptions about natural gender differences between men and women—in disposition and ability—justify both the ghettoization of women into lower-status and lower-paying jobs and the preference for men in higher-status and higher-paying jobs. When women do work in male-dominated jobs, managers and colleagues expect them to perform emotional labor, otherwise they might be considered cold and unapproachable.[12] Caring for others, however, can hinder women's abilities to do their jobs effectively and to be taken seriously by others. Caught between gender expectations to emotionally care for others (as women) and (masculine) occupational requirements to be decisive and emotionally removed, caring at work creates a catch-22 for women, whereby they are damned if they do and damned if they don't.

Jobs themselves are gendered.[13] They require bodies and behaviors we label masculine or feminine, which upholds the idea that it is men and women—not jobs—that are inherently different. As a female-dominated occupation, people come to see the way women nurse as a reflection of their sex rather than of the occupational requirement to care for others. Many consider men who do this job to be gender exceptions haunted by some sort of biological feminine inclination.[14] Men in care work do not make sense to us and others pressure them to explain themselves in socially acceptable ways and, for white men in particular, to take different, higher-status, and better paying jobs.[15] When men do nurse, they might find themselves lifting patients instead of bathing them, reinforcing rather than challenging gender dichotomies and the feminine characterization of the job.

Women who work in jobs that require care absolutely make sense to us. They meet socially agreed upon ideals for women and femininity, and in beauty work they operate by gender appropriate and occupationally required feeling rules. "Feeling rules," Arlie Hochschild explains, "guide emotion work by establishing the sense of entitlement or obligation that governs emotional exchanges."[16] Social guidelines about what, when, with whom, and how to feel often operate invisibly and are taken as natural reflections of personal, sex-linked, and even racially- and ethnically-linked predispositions. Feelings and expressions of care, though, are socially informed. As beauty providers working at Adonis and The Executive show, gendered feeling and touching rules differently shape how men and women do their jobs, as well as how they understand their relationships with clients and who they are as workers.

In her discussion of gendered organizations, sociologist Joan Acker leaves open the possibility of thinking about how sexuality interacts with class, race, and gender in organizations.[17] To theorize the gender of workplace actions, interactions, and relationships we must consider sexuality. Applying this approach, I find that women laboring within the heteronormative work cultures of Adonis and The Executive end up doing heterofeminine care work, by which emotional and physical care situates them as other women in their clients' lives.[18] Men who work at the salons show more flexibility in whether or not they intimately care for clients. Care work becomes disproportionately the responsibility of women, making women and their labor important sources of masculine ego and gender knowledge for male consumers.

The "Other Woman"

June had long black hair and wore tank tops to show off her sleeves of colorful floral tattoos. She seemed to enjoy talking about her clients and laughed as she exclaimed, "I'm the longest relationship they've had with a female, ever." Popular among The Executive's clients, June is always booked for appointments. While she provides clients with trendy haircuts, she also builds important relationships with them. These relationships are significant to June because she operates as a semi-entrepreneur. Commission and tips make up the bulk of the beauty workers' income,[19] and they are individually responsible for building a clientele. "If I want to do better, it's on me," Mirabel, a recent hire at the salon, said. Kendra also noted, "We develop friendships with our clients. . . . Obviously that's a good way to have clients come back to you." This "strategic friendliness" supports the women's bottom lines as they work to create a business within a business.[20] As June suggested, however, this relationship is important to clients for another reason—it provides them heterosocial friendship they might not otherwise get.

Men's relationships are often rife with competition, emotional detachment, and the collective sexual exploitation of women, and even nonhegemonic men often feel pressured by peers to live up to harmful definitions of masculinity that create barriers to intimacy.[21] Of course men can and do build close friendships with each other, but these are often relationships in which they do things with each other ("shoulder-to-shoulder" friendships) rather than have intimate conversations ("face-to-face" friendships).[22]

Women build friendships with more self-disclosure, intimacy, companionship, and loyalty.[23] Men often have fewer friends than women but do desire intimacy,[24] including "emotional support, disclosure, and having someone to take care of them."[25] Building friendships with their hairstylists or manicurists allows some men to find intimate and confidential relationships they otherwise lack. Despite social anxieties about the intersection of relationships and money, sociologist Viviana Zelizer assures us that intimacy is not a "fragile flower that withers on contact with money and economic self-interest." Within the growing service market, "Money cohabits regularly with intimacy, and even sustains it."[26]

"[Men] appreciate sitting in a chair and having a woman listen to them . . . they don't get that everyday," said Vicky. "I think they appreciate us more. . . . We're all friendly. I think they gravitate to us. They really enjoy being there. They feel like it's their place to come and just hang out with another woman and not feel guilty." Showing sympathy for men who juggle both family and work, Vicky believes men want to talk with women beauty workers because their wives or girlfriends may not listen to them. The idea that men might feel guilty for confiding in another woman suggests these relationships are indeed intimate and meaningful and reflects the stigma attached to nonsexual male-female relationships. In the vignette that opens this chapter, Isabel references Dean's wife, preventing (at least momentarily) sexual intimacy and allowing friendship to emerge. Men can also fold their interactions with the women into easily palatable discourses of utilitarianism; they have to have their hair cut, after all. This secrecy helps to protect men from backlash by their female partners, but it also makes many of the beauty providers see themselves as the "other woman" in their clients' lives.

The "other woman" identity helps women who groom men to claim meaningful roles as caregivers. This feeling of significance corroborates my earlier research where men talked about women hairstylists as providing them "another kind of relationship that is really important."[27] Some of the clients I interviewed indeed described themselves as having friendships with the women who cut their hair. Many of them said that they would nonetheless find a new provider or perhaps even a new salon if they were not happy with their haircut, manicure, or body wax. To these men, the women are replaceable as both coiffeurs and confidantes. Salons, after all, are packed with women who are expected to groom men physically and emotionally with little reciprocity. Despite, or perhaps because of this lack of reciprocity, workers' emotional labor has a different meaning for them than for their clients.

Caring becomes gendered as women end up with the responsibility of making men feel like men while they have their hair done or their nails buffed. By doing heteromasculinizing ego work the women attempt to make the men feel special.[28] Isabel explained that her clients "love to feel number one; they love to feel that they're special. . . . They love to hear that they're important in your life, even though they're not your husband or your boyfriend." If the men feel like they are personally important to the women, then they may come to the salon more regularly for appointments. To make men feel special, Isabel compliments their appearances and tells them she made time in her schedule especially for them. So while the women see themselves as the other woman in their clients' lives, Isabel believes the men likewise want to feel as if they are second only to their stylists' husbands or boyfriends.

The implication of intimacy within the worker-client exchange creates a potentially sexualized relationship, one that is characterized by emotional pleasure and physical exchange. Like Isabel, many of the women doing hair or even booking appointments at The Executive praise men on how they look. If men complain about their graying roots or receding hairline, the women assure them that their hair is not thinning too badly, and that gray hair is "sexy" on a man. Of course not all women believe their balding clients should feel confident about their lack of hair. They instead enact emotional labor by quelling their true feelings and purposefully bolstering their clients' egos. This ego work supports the salon's heterosexualized brand image and brings to life corporate promises to consumers that the women perform heterofeminine labor. Although sixty-year-old Martha doesn't see herself as heterosexually attractive as her younger female colleagues, she does believe her clients put more stock in her compliments than in their wives': "Even if the wife has said to them that morning, 'That shirt looks good on you,' and then I say it to them in the afternoon, I think it means more when I say it to them than the wife."

Women beauty workers serve-up masculinizing emotional labor to men in a way the male stylists do not. One online reviewer of a men's salon noted that "female affirmations" about how "great" his hair and skin looked after his appointment made him a satisfied customer. "There might be something to this place . . . I am trending [*sic*] toward four stars," he said. It is not simply female attention that makes men feel good, but attention from straight women. In chapter 3, I developed a framework for understanding how women's heterosexual identities are organizationally mobilized to create a heterosexual brand image and consumer experience. As part of this consumer experience, heterosexuality is not only privileged in these salons but also shapes the care work that masculinizes clients. By taking on the role of the doting other woman, the workers become complicit in—and capitalize on—heteronormativity at the same time they erase their individuality and deploy the female gaze.

The women working at Adonis and The Executive become stand-ins for all women. They explained that clients rely on them as gender experts, providing men with relationship advice and helping them to interpret the emotions of their wives and girlfriends. Clients want to know how women really think. To these men, the women told me, they have unique insight into the female species. Ruth, who had recently left her family's nail salon to forge her own career at The Executive, said that clients "want to know the low-down about women, the inside scoop." "We're girls," Mirabel said. So, "maybe if they're having a problem with a girl or something . . . we know the issues." Men, they reported, want advice on what characteristics women look for in men and what sorts of gifts women like. "Like, we have a lot of guys who are like, 'I don't know what to buy for my wife, it's my anniversary.' Or 'I was thinking to do this, what do you think she's gonna feel?'" said Isabel. In these situations, the women act as sources of gender knowledge for men who are uncertain about how to express affection for their wives or girlfriends. Helping to mediate men's relationships with other women, the stylists, nail technicians, estheticians, and even receptionists perform care work that extends beyond the walls of the salons to impact their clients' personal lives. They serve as clients' heterofeminine confidantes, providing men emotional support and a supposedly generic female opinion on all things related to women, while not being their wives or girlfriends. This role of gender expert naturalizes differences by framing women as plugged into some sort of biological female database of information.

"Guy Time"

Short with dark hair, Joshua wears trendy graphic t-shirts and canvas pants with Converse sneakers. He is the only licensed barber at Adonis, and one of two men who work there. When I asked him how he got into hair, he described the immensely meaningful relationships he forms with clients. As a youth minister, he values opportunities to help others and especially enjoys mentoring young men. Barbering, he told me, is one of those rare jobs that put men into close contact with each other. Cutting men's hair is an opportunity to care, he explained; and while he recognized that talking to clients is a tertiary aspect of the salon experience for many clients, it also allows him to get to know, listen to, and give advice to other men. The women say men prefer to confide in a female stylist, but Joshua explained: "For men to go in and see a guy, I think it could be for the idea of just having guy time." He challenges the idea that men's relationships have to be characterized by emotional detachment and instead embraces and enjoys the feeling rules of a feminized job that entails caring.

Joshua is an exception since guy time looks different for the other men working at Adonis and The Executive. He embraces doing hair precisely because it allows him to participate in care work and to foster platonic yet close relationships with other men.

Ryan and Randy do not invest in intimate relationships with their clients that are rooted in listening to their personal problems or providing them with life advice. They deemphasize the feeling rules of beauty work in favor of larger cultural expectations that men maintain emotionally distant relationships with each other. During my interview with Ryan, he avoided eye contact with me and stumbled through his explanation of the sort of relationships he builds with the men in his chair. This deemphasized approach to interacting with clients is reflected in how Ryan physically interacts with them. Joshua might hug a client "hello," but Ryan exhibits conventional masculine interactions by greeting his clients with a "Hi, dude!" and a handshake. Investing in the feeling rules that organize beauty work as intimate care work, Joshua reveals his interest in practicing intimacy-motivated emotional labor and challenges conventional ideas about just who can care. This investment in care work is a choice for Joshua, and risks emasculating both him and his clients, since masculinized feeling rules constrain men's intimacy with one another in many spaces. Joshua argues that some men are willing to confront these risks in order to secure a brotherly confidante, and in a place that offers both private dyadic worker-client interactions and a utilitarian service, the men's salon might be one of the safest places to do so.

Organizational cultures and job requirements shape how employees behave,[29] but people can and do make decisions about how to interpret gender scripts at work. Guy time for Joshua captures beauty providers' occupationally sanctioned and organizationally approved ability to talk with clients about their personal problems. For men who professionally groom other men, guy time can also mean avoiding dealing directly with men's emotions and instead involve bonding over more stereotypically masculine behavior, such as the sexual objectification of women. "Men feel more comfortable talking with other men about sexual indiscretions. They don't talk to me about that," explained Bridget, who waxes clients and shores up their nails. Having overheard Randy carry on tawdry conversations with some of his clients at The Executive, Bridget said that men "sit there talking about women they slept with, and these are men with wives. And [they say], 'What happens in Vegas stays in Vegas.'" Randy nods along to his clients' excited, detailed descriptions of hot dates and sexual encounters with women, she told me. Collectively objectifying women is a popular practice among boys and men that reveals more about the misogyny upon which men's relationships and identities are built than about their actual sexual desires. Friends and family might see men who go to the hair salon as consuming a homosexual aesthetic,[30] but this risk is mitigated by guy time that emphasizes heterosexuality as masculinity.

Collectively sexualizing women is prevalent even in environments were people might otherwise presume the "new man" is emerging.[31] The hair salon is often depicted in the news as a site for the production and persistence of a new kind of masculinity, and white, well-to-do men suggest they are more progressive than blue-collar men for going to a salon rather than to Supercuts or a barbershop.[32] The "new man," however, is a problematic concept because it emphasizes temporal gender displays over structural positions of power, and it ignores how men's behaviors such as beautifying can be a sign of power and does little to unsettle raced, classed, and gender hierarchies. The new man is more ideological than actual, with theories on hybridization suggesting such a conceptualization is an example of how hegemony—or ideologies and discourses assuring the dominance of some—is dialectical.[33] Dominant masculinities are reconstituted through-out time by drawing from other visible, more marginalized groups such as women and gay men so as to appear counter-hegemonic, when in real-ity this hybridization is a "strategy for the reproduction of patriarchy" and other unequal power structures.[34]

The need to talk about women's bodies, brag about heterosexual con-quests, and otherwise reduce women to sexual objects demonstrates just how masculine identities and status are built at the expense of women. So, while men appear to engage a new and progressive masculinity by consum-ing beauty practices, they use misogynist heterosexual discourses as tools to approach masculinity vis-à-vis heterosocial interactions (see chapter 3). This is despite the idea that young white men are able to access more flex-ible masculinities without harm to their social status.[35] Aggie, a magenta-haired stylist at The Executive, suggested clients might prefer women stylists because they don't make the men feel as if they have failed at doing masculinity. When men do request an appointment with Randy—one of three licensed barbers at The Executive—she said it is because men "are a little more crass and just want to talk about tits and ass all the time." Some men, she said, "just don't like talking to women in general," because they might be socially uncomfortable around or harbor hostile feelings toward women.

The gendered feeling rules of beauty work, which require care, and larger masculine feeling rules, which constrain men's cultivation of intimate het-erosocial interactions, clash at Adonis and The Executive. And so, for men employed at the salons, this gendered feature of their job is not rigid. There are different pathways for men to forge relationships with their clients. But how might Ryan and Randy still provide socio-psychological support to the men in their chairs? While their relationships with clients are not built on the same sort of emotional labor Joshua and the women perform, Ryan and Randy nonetheless do masculinizing ego work by supporting men's heterosexual identities. Maintaining emotional distance from their clients and engaging in hetero-aggressive banter, they manage clients' associations with potentially emasculating beauty regimes and their own discomfort with a feminized job. They deemphasize emotional occu-pational mandates and skills, including deference and sensitivity. Ryan, who holds a cosmetology license, made sure to tell me that he is planning to enroll in barber college. Barber college will train him in straight-razor shaves, but it also acts as a tie to a more historically male-dominated occupation that allows him to distinguish himself from the women alongside whom he works. At the same time, it is not clear how Ryan and Randy really feel about their clients. Perhaps, like Joshua, they too long to create close relationships with other men but suppress these feelings to make clients heterosexually comfortable. Or perhaps they have no interest in building more emotionally sympathetic relationships with clients. Either way, systems of gender and heterosexuality structure their emotional labor so that it looks different from the women's while similarly supporting clients' social identities as privileged straight men.

The Race and Gender of Listening to Men

Emotional labor at The Executive becomes clearly racialized when considering the experiences of Antonio, a thirty-five-year-old Mexican immigrant shoe shiner, who is the salon's longest standing employee. I never met Elliot, the salon's other shoe shiner, because he worked part time and irregular hours. As a black man, he and Antonio exemplify how the gender of care work is filtered through race and ethnicity. Shoe shining has a racialized history as an entrepreneurial opportunity for black men that subordinates them to whites.[36] In fact, "Distinct traces of a racial-caste system shaped the minority-business community throughout most of the twentieth century,"[37] and shoe shining is an occupation by which black and Latino men have long supported the classed embodiments and entitled feelings of wealthy white men. The image of a well-dressed white man sitting in a raised leather chair with a man of color spit-shining his shoes celebrates the existing inequalities among men, the gendered racialization of different sorts of body work, and the racialization of so called dirty work.

Antonio walks around The Executive with unparalleled focus. He doesn't stop to chat with the stylists or receptionists, and he is constantly moving, as his job turns janitorial when there are no shoe shine clients. For Antonio, the most "disgusting" part of his job is when he picks up dirty towels covered in clients' hair and sweat. His responsibility for this work, combined with his immigrant and ethnic status, limits Antonio's interactions with clients. He claimed to like it this way, telling me that he prefers when clients drop off their shoes with him while they get a haircut. The complimentary black sandals available to clients in the Locker Room make this possible: men can simply pick up their freshly polished shoes on their way out of the salon. At times I saw men drop off entire bags of shoes for Antonio to shine. This consumer convenience threatens to make Antonio's work invisible to clients, but it also allows him to minimize interpersonal work.

In his nine years working at The Executive, Antonio had not become comfortable listening and responding to the intimate details of clients' lives. There are men who prefer to sit high up on the shoe shine chair, reading the *L.A. Times* while Antonio kneels, head down at their feet to polish away the scuffs on their leather shoes. These men, he said, sometimes divulge personal information that he rather not know. While clients do not seem to enact the same sort of intimate relationships with Antonio as they do with the female stylists, they will nonetheless confess their worries to him. But where the women provide men advice, Antonio remains largely silent. His status as an ethnic immigrant is particularly salient at the salon, and so clients might not expect him to relate to or be able to provide them advice on their white middle-class troubles. He is also outside of these men's social networks, allowing clients to feel secure confiding in him. Antonio serves as an obliged sounding board for these men, and they expect him to either not understand what they are saying or to safeguard their personal information.

Clients' interactions with Antonio secure and sustain class-privileged white masculinity. While gender inequality is popularly conceptualized as male dominance/female subordination, intersectional analyses of race, class, sexuality, and gender reveal that gender hierarchies exist among men and among women. White clients who purchase shoe shines are directly connected to a racist history in which men of color perform obsequious reproductive labor. Feminist theory uses "reproductive labor" to refer to the domestic work of women who care for the home and family, and thus who reproduce the husband as a capitalist worker.[38] Antonio similarly reproduces the white-collar worker by maintaining the dress shoes of men in accounting, advertising, software, engineering, and law. His relationship to the beauty workers was similarly shaped by ethnicity. While the women performed heterosexual aesthetic labor and care work that made them deferential to clients, they also moved around the salon taking for granted that Antonio would clean up after them. In this way, race and ethnicity intersect with gender to make Antonio subordinate and often invisible to clients and other employees.

HEARTS AND HANDS

The body is central to work. Just because physically demanding industry labor no longer monopolizes the U.S. economy doesn't mean that work "no longer require[s] hands."[39] Changing patterns in work have resulted in the increased commodification of the body, so that corporations now rely on workers' bodies to not only produce goods but to also act as commodities. Work is obviously embodied in that it takes bodies to do work, but some jobs also shape or remake workers' appearances: male construction workers develop weathered hands as a sign of blue-collar masculinity and retail workers fit the aesthetics of their corporate brand (see chapter 3).[40] Jobs such as beauty work require employees to physically manipulate and maintain the bodies of others.[41] Considering the different ways bodies work—as well as under what conditions and to what ends—helps us to more fully understand how inequalities inform contemporary meanings and experiences of work. Because, "[A]lthough everyone has a body, not everyone has the same relation to its economic and symbolic significance."[42]

Emerging research on bodies at work build on Hochschild's scholarship of emotions in the service economy.[43] Workers' appearances and physical interactions with customers are additional, not replacement, foci for the study of service work. Social relations are reflected in and shape human bodies and human feelings, and so beauty work is an excellent case for exploring the complicated and meaningful relationship between hearts and hands at work. Kang's study of Korean nail technicians serves as the most comprehensive empirical effort to bring the two together. Focusing largely on the requirements to labor on the bodies of others, Kang highlights how social stratification funnels some people into bodily labor and other people into consumer roles. "[C]ertain women," she says, "benefit from the intimate body and emotional labor of other women at great costs to both those who serve them and the goals of more egalitarian relations."[44] But what about men? Do they too benefit from the emotional and physically intimate labor of women? Of other men? Systems of gender and heterosexuality result in different feeling rules for the men and women working at Adonis and The Executive, and this is also true in regards to the touching rules that script their physical interactions with clients. Touching rules, I argue, inform the emotional labor of workers and reveal the dialectical relationship between "words" and "actions" when serving-up care to male beauty consumers.

Touching rules are socially, culturally, and contextually specific norms enabling and constraining who can touch whom, how, and under what conditions, as well as how people are supposed to feel about this touch. Touching rules highlight the importance of bodies and bodily collisions in service work and allows for a theoretical emphasis on social norms around bodies that can help us to understand touch in various contexts. Like feeling rules, touching rules at Adonis and The Executive differ for female and male workers—sometimes operating independently, other times together. These differences shape the political economy of workers' bodies, whereby the emotions and bodies of differently sexed and gendered workers become unequally commercialized.

A Woman's Touch

Hair and nail industry reports note that both men and women are increasingly interested in a pampered consumer experience,[45] and workers believe pampering is a key reason men choose Adonis and The Executive for their haircuts and manicures. Over and over again, women told me the shampoo plays an especially big role in men's satisfaction with the salons' services. "It relaxes them," said Joanne, a forty-one-year-old stylist at The Executive who had worked in hair for almost nineteen years. "They've been stressed out and I've had many times where as soon as they get down there and I rub their neck, they're like, 'Oh! I needed that!' It's a huge, huge deal." Adonis once had a plumbing problem, "Something happened in the back alley," Patricia, a twenty-eight-year-old Latina stylist, told me. "Plumbing, no bueno with the sinks." The salon was open, but stylists could not shampoo clients' hair. They instead "had to just do spray-downs for the clients." Men were "up in arms," she said. "My clients were like, 'Oh, I look forward to the hot towel treatment! I look forward to my scalp massage! You owe me next time, an even longer one!'"

Delivering men a physically pampering shampoo with scalp massage or a hot towel facial involves the careful and intimate touch of women beauty workers. "I really like having women wash my hair, to be quite honest, especially with long fingernails," said Noah, my friend who introduced me to Adonis. Men working at Adonis and The Executive did not describe digging their nails deep into clients' hair, nor did they express pride in moaning clients or talk about being jealous of other stylists who appear to touch clients so effortlessly. The men have to touch their clients to do their jobs, but this touch is framed and constrained by presumptions of clients' homophobia and discomfort with homosocial physical exchanges. Noah, for example, went on to tell me that he would be less comfortable having a man shampoo his hair: "I wouldn't be as relaxed. I don't think it's an overly sexual thing, but there's definitely a sexual element to it."

Caring for clients via purposeful, physical caressing falls on the shoulders of women beauty providers. Touching and pampering is considered by beauty work scholars to be more raced and gendered than sexual,[46] yet women working at these men's salons described the heterosexual pleasure they ostensibly provide men when performing a deep scalp massage or a creamed foot rub. In fact, when I asked the women why it is they believe clients might prefer a woman hairstylist to a man, their number one reason was: they "want to be touched by a woman." Their second: wanting to talk to a woman.

"They're like, 'I just need your touch. I'm single. I need a woman to touch me," said Gabrielle. She leaned toward me and intensely waved her hands around as she described the different ways that she saw her interactions with clients as heterosexual. She continued to impersonate her clients: "'I just need a woman to touch my hair. Play with it a little bit, relax my skull, make me focus again and then I go to work again and I'm feeling better.'" She was adamant that men want a woman's touch, and the men's salon is a safe place in which men can seek out the touch of young, attractive women. The women proposed that this care comes not only from acting as heterofeminine confidantes to men but also from providing men pleasurable touch. They again become "other women" in their interactions with clients, providing men the physical intimacy they might desire but do not get elsewhere. Touch is an important part of the human experience, and the women understand this. They see touch as a human necessity, and the fact that they can provide this physical contact fills what many of the workers see as gaps in clients' heterosexual relationships with women. They cast wives and girlfriends as having the power to deny or provide men with physical intimacy—an idea that overlooks both the fact that men often exercise entitlement to women's bodies and sexualities and that they themselves lack the power to deny their clients.

Isabel explained that hairdressers are the only other people besides wives who are allowed to touch men in intimate ways. "The wife and the hairdresser, those are the only two people that can touch their hair." She suggested that touching rules dictated by larger norms around heterosexuality and monogamy mean many men are starved of touch. As a stylist, though, she is in a position to ruffle her fingers through men's hair and to massage their scalps. Women believe they serve as temporary, surrogate girlfriends for some of their clients.[47] After all, being the other woman means being physically, not just emotionally, intimate with clients. But providing tactile pleasure to men within the confines of high-service beauty work is not straightforward, rather, it involves managing the potential feminizing effect of pampering on men. And these women evoke a masculinizing emotional labor to accomplish this.

Women's beauty shops or hair salons are places for pampering and leisure. Women might spend two or three hours there having their hair assessed, shampooed, cut, dyed, straightened, curled, moisturized, and styled, and perhaps they throw in a mani or a pedi. Well-to-do white men have also historically sought out pampering at the barbershop, which used to provide them a bevy of corporeally relaxing and enhancing services.[48] In more recent history, however, men lack such places. Employees at Adonis and The Executive contend that the sorts of places men often have their hair cut, like Supercuts or Great Clips, turn over clients too quickly to provide a leisurely and luxurious experience, and that barbershops lack pampering services. "Women," Corey, owner and sole stylist of a competing men's salon, said, "[are] used to being pampered. Men are not." While men might go to a women's salon to access elaborate, pleasurable shampoos,[49] Corey believes men also feel like and are treated by stylists as "second-class citizens" in these places. Contemporary salons like his own are designed for men, offering clients the chance to be "pampered like women" while also being "catered to" as men.

Since men might desire but are often inexperienced with pampering, the beauty workers at Adonis and The Executive worry their clients will feel uncomfortable being touched during services. In an effort to create repeat customers the women learn to touch in particular ways. *Touching right* highlights just how gender ideologies translate into precise and appropriate ways of physically engaging others. Touching rules help employees to touch right, according to their occupational regimes and the organizational culture of their workplaces. This touch, for the women working at Adonis and The Executive, means providing men with intimate, caring tactile exchanges that do not strain worker-client interactions and that do not make men feel emasculated. To accomplish these goals, the women follow two golden rules when touching clients: appear confident and do not feminize.

To make clients comfortable with being touched, the stylists have to be self-assured in touching the men. "If you touch them in a way, they can sense that you're uncomfortable. So you have to just be confident," Vicky said. As a new hire who was still learning how to touch right, she highlighted the sort of socio-psychological conditioning in which women participate to become "touchy-feely." The way stylists touch men, Vicky explained, can "make or break" clients' experiences at The Executive, and by extension the stylists' tips. Stylists can't hesitate to "get in there and do the job," even when they are appalled by some clients' greasy hair. This requires stylists to swallow their feelings of disgust in order to provide the right kind of touch that makes men feel physically pampered. This emotional labor helps women to provide a touch that feels natural and leisurely to clients, and clients need to think the women are enjoying touching them. "Guys will freak out" if the women appear rushed or don't dig into their scalps. "If you just did a quick shampoo, whatever, it shows that you don't care," Mirabel told me. "But if you're giving just an extra minute or two to give a massage, they're like, 'OK, this person isn't rushing me out of here. They want to take their time.'" Even in cosmetology school, instructors taught the beauty workers to touch clients in very specific ways: slowly and steadily so as to appear in control of their touch. Touching right is a cultivated skill performed convincingly through emotional control so that the women appear competent and put clients at ease.

Beauty workers at Adonis and The Executive walk a fine line between providing clients with a luxurious, class-privileged experience of beauty and larger feminine associations of pampering. They are careful to not make touch feel "feminine" to men. "You have to pamper guys in a masculine way," Corey told me. As a gay stylist, he has an incentive to make men feel comfortable with same-sex touch in his salon, but he also believes it's his job to initiate men into the pampering culture of male grooming. Aggie exemplified the thought beauty workers put into touch on the job. She told me that when guiding men to her station: "If I'm touching them, it'll be on the back of their shoulder. It's not like I'm grabbing them by the waist and bringing them in." She laughed, imagining what this might look like and how clients might react. Of course it is men who tend to exhibit control over women's bodies by grabbing them at the waist and guiding them around, and so touching men in this way would undermine social scripts of gender expectations and power.

If you are not comfortable touching others, then doing hair or nails is not for you. Touching others should come naturally to beauty workers, women told me. Dividing beauty workers from non-beauty workers, they claimed that grooming others is a natural occupational fit for women like them—who are innate nurturers—and it is the ability to touch others confidently that situates beauty work as a "calling." They understand that cultural taboos around touch make people curious about their work. Connie, a twenty-four-year-old stylist at Adonis, said, "Some people think, 'You're touching them. Isn't that weird?'" But the women explained away any hesitation about this aspect of their job by claiming to be "naturally touchy." Several women attempted to prove this by telling me stories in which they were caught stroking strangers' hair at bars or restaurants; and Emily, a short, peppy twenty-one-year-old stylist at Adonis, demonstrated this by leaning in to touch me. "We're all like that," she said. "We're like, 'OK!' and you just touch their arm [rubs my left arm], and you're like 'Oh!' and you touch their hair [sweeps my bangs out of my face] . . . you're touching people all day, touching people's faces. . . . I've always been like a friendly, huggy person. I've gotten more like that with this [job]."

The women expressed pride in their ability to naturally and comfortably touch their clients, and described just how unique and important this aspect of their job is. "I don't think in any other job you really have that touch," Elsie, a twenty-three-year-old stylist at Adonis, told me. "I feel like people need that in their lives, with everything, even going to the doctor's it's an uncomfortable feeling. This is the only place, the beauty industry, that you actually get to be touched and relaxed and pampered." Bridget agreed, saying, "As humans we don't touch each other enough," and so men can fulfill their need for tactile care at the salon. Elsie not only explains the importance of touch, but also conceptualizes touch as having different meanings and visceral effects depending on where and by whom people are touched. The doctor's office provides a sterilized form of touch that is not meant to fulfill desires for gratifying tactile care; it is not even meant to be medicinal. To be pleasurable, touch needs to be both relaxing and pampering, and beauty workers are perfectly situated to provide this. From this perspective, Elsie and other women at Adonis and The Executive occupy a privileged job, whereby they provide valuable touch to their clients. Touch is more than simply a work requirement; it is adopted as a skill and a joy, providing the women a sense of job satisfaction. "It's just nice to give that to somebody, a relaxation, a healing," explained Connie.

By expressing a deep sense of pleasure in their ability to help clients meet the human need for touch, these women gave me the impression that they are "paid to play."[50] That is, their jobs don't feel like work because their ability to touch is seemingly natural and they enjoy what they do. Of course the rhetoric about women as naturally "touchy-feely," as Vicky described it, veils the fact that beauty providers have to learn to touch. They learn touching rules: who they can touch, how, and under what conditions. Because women are culturally cast as naturally caring, their expressions of emotional and physical care often go unnoticed or are taken-for-granted as effortless and signs of their innate femininity. Physically caring for others requires a lot of energy, though, and some stylists said they are disgusted when men come in with greasy, dirty hair. Nail technicians do not love clipping men's dirty nails or scraping off men's calluses. So although describing themselves as simply "like that"—naturally touchy—it became clear the women learned to appear confortable with intimate cross-gender touch at work.

Male Stylists and the Suppression of Touch

Cultural scripts that inform hegemonic masculinity constrain men's emotional and physical intimacy with others. It is not manly to express emotions, and so hugging another man becomes sissy and closeness with a female friend must be an expression of sexual desire. But there are some contexts in which men can touch other men without coming under suspicion of being gay. On the football field and in the locker room men might playfully smack each others' rears. Sport is a masculine institution that protects male athletes from stigma, so much so that sports have served as a sort of closet for gay men.[51] The hair salon and the practice of beauty work, however, make suspect the sexual identities of male beauty workers. The trope of the effeminate gay male stylist is well known. And even though barbering is a male dominated occupation, male barbers working at Adonis and The Executive risk feminization by their association with a high-service salon.

They aren't cutting hair in a typical barbershop, popularly characterized as a small, dated, no-frills space with automobile magazines piled in the corner. They similarly are not working in a high-end hipster barbershop. Barbers aren't known for providing pampering touch, anyway; they don't massage their clients' scalps, provide facials, or lather up men's fingers in preparation for a detailed manicure. But at Adonis and The Executive, this sort of touch is built into the luxurious salon-going experience and thus the work regimes of the salons' employees, helping the owners to distinguish their salons as new places for "men who care." So how do the men working at these salons navigate the tensions between cultural expectations that men do not touch other men and occupational expectations that they carefully and intimately touch clients?

Heterosexuality and homophobia—as tools for masculine expression—inform the touching rules of both women and men at these salons, albeit differently. Men and women working in the same place and who hold the same jobs do not do the same work. Just as the men might avoid taking on the intimate role of hairapist, they also avoid touching their clients as much as possible. The touching rules by which the men operate are shaped by expectations that they develop socially acceptable homosocial interactions with their clients. After all, Randy, Ryan, and Joshua identify as straight and the salons are in the business of providing a heteromasculinizing consumer experience—despite clients' sexual identities. Consequently, while the women I interviewed explained that men enjoy being touched by women, the men added that clients sometimes avoid male stylists altogether. When the topic of touch came up in my interview with Ryan, he said, "some guys want a chick workin' on 'em, either because they're homophobic or they may want—maybe they just want a cute girl workin' on 'em or somethin.'"

Julie, a twenty-year-old receptionist at The Executive, said that often times when men schedule their appointments they request women. She believes men are aware that getting their hair done or their cuticles clipped requires at least some touch, and that they might feel "weird" being touched by another man. "I would say, for some men, it just creeps them out to have their head rubbed by another man. [Laughs]. Whatever it may be, that just kind of seems weird to them." Noah reinforced this, saying that he would not want to have his hair done by a man because, while the haircut is not blatantly sexual, "It's a pretty intimate space. It's your head!" Rea, twenty-three-year-old stylist at Adonis, insinuated that some clients might indeed feel uncomfortable having another man cut their hair, and for this reason it is difficult to retain male employees. "We've tried to have more male stylists, and it either just wouldn't work out or whatever."

Assuming clients are heterosexual makes invisible the salons' gay clientele and overlooks the sexualization of the male stylists. Joshua believes that some men at Adonis like to have their hair cut by a barber because it is what they know, since they may have grown up going to a barber and so are comfortable with this setup. Going to a stylist is just "too gay" for some men, one of the women at The Executive told me. At the same time, women cutting hair at Adonis sometimes laughed as they described men who request appointments with "pretty boy" Ryan. Patricia smiled at the idea that Ryan has to deal with clients who find him sexually attractive. "Even some of my clients are like, 'He's so hot! How do you work with him?'" Ryan, however, doesn't find this quite as funny. "I just do my job," he told me. Avoiding eye contact with me, he explained: "Some people ask me, 'Don't you think they're gonna hit on you?' I don't care. Whatever. Because I know that—I know what my motives are, and I feel like I'm pretty confident in who I am." Ryan avoids appearing homophobic, but he also does not embrace his sexual appeal to clients, which might raise questions about his own sexuality.

Ryan went on to tell me that while his cosmetology school instructor encouraged students to touch clients in ways that create a pleasurable experience for them, he has since learned to tone down this touch. For this reason, high-service bodily labor looks different for men who groom other men, and thus men who have their hair cut and styled by Ryan get a different sort of physical experience at Adonis. He shampoos men's hair before a cut but generally avoids slow, methodic movements where he digs his fingers into their hair to massage their scalps. His shampoos are often quicker than those of the women with whom he works. He claims this is to avoid making his clients feel uncomfortable. Some women at The Executive noticed that their male colleagues followed occupational touching rules when Veronica first hired them but that as they become experienced in men's grooming, the way they perform their jobs changed. Joanne, Aggie, and Loretta, a nail technician, sat around the outdoor patio table during their break, talking about the ways Randy and a past male stylist, Matt, altered the way they shampoo clients:

JOANNE: Do Randy and Matt even massage their necks?

AGGIE: No, not really.

JOANNE: They don't really do it, because I think they're not comfortable doing it either. I don't know if that's it, if they're not comfortable or they're just concerned about the client being [uncomfortable].

LORETTA: I thought they did. Maybe they're just sensitive to ones they know don't want it. But I think the ones that are willing—

AGGIE: Yeah, Matt is very touchy, isn't he?

LORETTA: He used to be a lot more. I don't know what changed. But yeah, he used to spend a lot of time shampooing, but he doesn't anymore.

JOANNE: Maybe somebody—

LORETTA: I'll have to ask about that.

JOANNE: Maybe people were worried he's gay [Laughs].

The question remains: if clients are not comfortable being touched by a man, then why do they go to a male stylist or barber? By making appointments with a male stylist or barber, clients may not avoid being touched by another man, but they do avoid the potentially feminizing touch that accompanies pampering in a high-service salon. They can assure their associations with professional-class embodied consumer habits and access familiar interactions with a male barber—or at least a man they may presume to be a barber. Roxy, who had plans to open her own men's salon, said clients are surprised to find out she is a barber because they simply assume barbers are men and men are barbers.

Feminizing Pampering, Masculinizing Emotional Labor

Trish, who massages clients at Adonis, has given the confidante role she plays at work a lot of thought. "I get people that are practically strangers telling me very intimate things," she said. Over the years, people have told her "things that I know they wouldn't be telling other people." Unlike other women she works with, Trish doesn't consider herself to be a particularly nurturing person, but she finds that when men lay face down on her table, they make muffled confessions and sometimes even sob. The women explain this largely as a gendered connection with men, whereby men feel safe confiding in women. As they continued to reflect on their intimate interactions with clients and what it means to care for men at the salons, the women connected touch with clients' emotional release and with the emotional labor they perform at work.

Women's heterofeminine care work at Adonis and The Executive is, in part, a function of their occupational requirements to touch. They explained that developing a close, intimate relationship with men in their chairs begins with breaking larger touching rules that usually constrain physical interactions between strangers. Massaging a client's scalp, exfoliating his face, and rubbing his feet create a sense of trust between worker and client. This is particularly important when working with men, Isabel said, because, "Men are so hard to trust people. . . . So the key of them to trust you is touching." When done right, touching men will relax them, and as they relax, women told me, men divulge the intimate details of their lives. Jackie, Adonis's esthetician, said, "You connect with people on a different level because you're physically there with someone and you're touching them and you're talking to them and they just start spilling their guts." The women massage men's scalps, hands, and faces, and when clients begin to disclose personal information, the women listen. Even Corey noted that when he touches men, "the shield goes down and their mouth [sic] opens up and all this stuff starts coming out."

But how is this relationship between touch and talk gendered? Women, after all, also open up to their stylists. Does being gay allow Corey to care for men in ways different from the straight men working at Adonis and The Executive? Because cultural definitions of masculinity generally prohibit, or at least inhibit, tactile and emotional intimacy between men, the touch women provide at the salons might satiate men's need for physical contact. Connie, at Adonis, said, "When you get a massage, you need that. It's like a healing thing." Touch—it's a human need men might not get as often as women, who have more social space to hug and touch others. If the hair salon is the only other place besides heterosexual romantic relationships men can get touched by a woman, as workers attest, then both the beauty workers and the salon become important sources for a pleasurable tactile experience.

Pampering touch in the high-service men's salons upholds both the classed expectations of men who expect luxurious consumer experiences and the gendered experience of being cared for by women. At the same time, however, being pampered in hair salons and through beauty services is associated largely with women, and so stylists discussed having to use *masculinizing emotional labor* to manage this potentially feminizing touch. Touch and emotion rules work dialectically to protect masculinity.

Men who are not used to being physically pampered, or who struggle with its feminine associations, might be squeamish or unsure about the scalp massage that accompanies the shampoo or the hot towel service built into the mini-facial at Adonis. One online reviewer noted that "women go do the silly things they do" but that "it feels good to pamper yourself." Another said, "I am not accustomed to getting 'pampered like a lady,'" but then challenges men, "let's face it guys, why not??!!"

Women working at Adonis and The Executive assure men they are not facing potential emasculation by leaning their heads back in the sinks to enjoy a relaxing shampoo. They walk clients through services, describing to men what to expect during their appointments so that clients are not caught off guard when stylists whip out exfoliator to cleanse their faces. Patricia, a twenty-eight-year-old stylist at Adonis, said, "I explain it if it's a new client, 'We do the haircut, we do a hot towel treatment, that's a facial scrub. You just sit back and relax.' Most of 'em are just—and they've never had anybody touch them like that." Women not only initiate men into beauty and educate them on the intricacies of high-service beauty practices, they also manage men's feelings of apprehension about the gendered and sexualized meanings attached to these practices.

Stylists assure men that the facial and shampoo are not emasculating. They try to assuage men's anxieties by telling them it is not "gay" to have their scalp massaged. The women tell their clients that if they don't get over their fears then they will miss out on a "human" pleasure to which their wives and other men are privy. Degendering pampering services as something enjoyable to any person, the women attempt to soothe men's anxieties around these practices and to produce a sense of calm—and hopefully pleasure and loyalty—for clients. In this way, the women end up compensating for and reframing physically pleasurable and luxurious beauty service for men. This masculinizing emotional labor supports men's egos by undercutting the assumptions about the salon as a gendered institution and just who should be purchasing and enjoying salon services.

"Beauty is pain," goes the saying. The idea that women often consent to physical pain in order to achieve—or to approximate—beauty standards is well known. They corset their waists, pluck their eyebrows, perm their hair with harsh chemicals, and slip on heels that pinch their toes together.

But men are not supposed to feel pain, or at least not complain about pain: "Be a man!" "Boys don't cry!" "Shake it off!" Cultural definitions of men as "sturdy oaks" and of masculinity as void of "sissy stuff" encourage men to be tough guys, invulnerable and unemotional.[52] And so what does it mean when men yelp as beauty workers (or wives and girlfriends) pluck their eyebrows? Are they no longer real men?

Jackie explained that because waxing can hurt, she tries to turn men's expressions of pain into non-issues. Men might feel less manly not simply because they are having their backs, chests, or "bikini" areas waxed, but because they squirm in discomfort and yell out in protest when she applies hot wax and tears out their hair. She assures them, "Anyone would be hurt getting waxed. It's not so much, 'Oh, you're a guy, it shouldn't hurt. It should tickle.'" Jackie reveals the emotional labor involved when waxing men, especially since this sort of touch might induce pain or fear of pain not conventionally compatible with hegemonic masculinity. She and other workers use emotional labor to masculinize men's experiences of physical pampering, and to make the salons safe spaces in which men can consume beauty services and reveal fears without having to renounce their masculinity. She lets them know that there is nothing wrong with or unmasculine about them because they are uneasy about being waxed or because they flinch when she yanks the carpets from their backs.

CONCLUSION

Intimacy and friendship is characterized by reciprocity. There are degrees of intimacy, though, and many of the men who frequent Adonis and The Executive secure emotionally supportive and physically pleasurable relationships with women without having to reciprocate or otherwise "sacrifice their own self-interest."[53] This does not mean men are selfish or that they don't care for their stylists, manicurists, or estheticians. But in a society that conflates hegemonic masculinity with the suppression of close emotional and physical exchanges with others—and in a workplace that relies on women to be caregivers—these men are able to fulfill their desires for confidential and heterosexual intimacy without having to compromise masculine feeling or touching rules.[54]

The women create esteem-building definitions of their work that reject the frivolousness of vanity. Clients, however, do not have to protect their status while they enjoy a luxurious shampoo because cultural demands on women's emotions and occupational and institutional demands on women's bodies do this for them. The production of care via talk and touch at Adonis and The Executive subordinates women workers to male clients and boosts men's class privileges and masculine egos. Men—especially white men—are used to their interests being at the center of attention and conversation,[55] and this entitlement supports both the invisibility of women's work and the biologized notion of women's propensity to care.

Tensions between feminized occupational requirements to care and larger masculine expectations to avoid intimacy allow Ryan and Randy to escape institutionalized requirements to forge intimate relationships. Expressing discomfort with the feminized character of his job, Ryan, who held a cosmetology license, stressed to me that he was planning to attend barber college and used the title of "barber" to differentiate himself from his female colleagues and to avoid the intimate care work built into doing hair. Scholarship shows that black barbers care for their patrons as mentors, provide monetary loans, and talk with men about health issues. In the black barbershop, barbers and clients similarly experience large-scale and everyday racial subordination, and so they share interests that bind them in a unique way. The white professional clients at Adonis and The Executive occupy privileged social locations that keep them from needing the advice of their barber. Men's homosocial pampering touch is also constrained, relieving men of the same sort of physical labor and masculinizing emotional labor the women do. This raises questions about men's work identities and job satisfaction. Could they create naturalized identities as beauty workers? Would they want to? How are they rewarded or hurt by constraints on care work? These questions speak to the way gendered feeling rules and touching rules both reflect the hegemonic positions of men in the salons and come with costs to men's emotive freedoms.

5 · "WE'RE MEN'S WOMEN"

Occupational Choice Narratives of Sameness and Difference

"Men are great," Martha said. Having attended barbering college in her early fifties, she told me, "It's very low-drama, very easy, relaxed. . . . They're easy. It's easy for me. But I've always had men friends and when I was in high school I had guy friends. And I have five sons, so it works for me." When I asked Martha why she applied to The Executive, she said that she is "relaxed being around them" and explained that working with men seemed like a natural choice for someone who has always had "guy friends." She did not want me getting the impression that she "totally understands" men, but she does consider herself to have been a "tomboy" as a child. Describing herself as "more like a man," Martha reminisced about accompanying her brother to the barbershop in her younger years: "When I took my brother, I like[d] the smells. I liked the guys sitting reading the papers, joking around. I just thought it was awesome."

Martha described women in contrast to men as overly emotional and demanding about their hair. Although she had never worked with women clients, she was sure it would be challenging: "Being in beauty shops, for me, I saw—as you're getting your hair colored, I'd see women going, 'I want hair like this,' and I've heard the stylist say, 'Well, that's a neat style, however, with your face shape and your hair type—' 'No! I want *this* style!' Mad. Then they'll do it, and I'll see the finished product and it'll look exactly like what they described, and the woman going, 'I'm not paying you.'" Her personal anecdotes—from observing other women when she has her own hair done—made it sound as if cutting and styling women's hair would be absolute misery. "Oh man, I'm not going through that. No way!" she exclaimed.

The idea that men are more friendly, easygoing, and fun to work with and be around than women dominated the *occupational choice narratives* of women who worked at The Executive. They deployed explanations to quell the unease of people who might be otherwise suspicious about women who work at a salon that requires them to have constant and intimate contact with men. The women forged gender identities at the same time they explained why they work at a men's salon: "I'm a tomboy" and "We're men's women," they told me. By aligning themselves with men, these women participated in a process that sociologist Patricia Yancey Martin refers to as "practicing gender."[1] Informed by dramaturgical notions of "doing gender,"[2] Martin argues that gender is created through everyday "sayings and doings," whereby people project masculinities and femininities through discourse and behavior. How people practice gender is contextual in that they draw from locally available gender conceptions to forge identities and relationships in a given situation. Drawing from the ways masculinity and femininity are framed in their workplaces, women at Adonis and The Executive wove different stories about their decisions to work with men, and about just what kind of women they are.

Women employed at The Executive practiced gender via discourses of sameness and difference. They emphasized personal traits and tastes that they associated with masculinity, such as casualness and noncompetitive relationships with friends, and they vehemently rejected women as "real bitches." By carving out identities as exceptional women who are "more like men," they disrupt static ideas that sex (being male or female) dictates gender (i.e., expressions of masculinity or femininity) while also essentializing differences between men and women. They trade on misogyny by deploying sexist discourses that associate them with men and masculinity and devalue women as a group.[3] In a place where there is no room for femininity, even the women's gender identities celebrate men and masculinity. Women employed at Adonis, conversely, did not generate occupational choice narratives or gender identities that aligned them more closely with men than with other women. Unlike women at The Executive, many of the stylists at Adonis do not spend every day with men. They work part time at Adonis's sister salon, Bonita, where they snip, dye, and style women's hair. They expressed a deep sense of appreciation for working on and interacting with women, and they enjoy the range of creativity allowed at Bonita and talking with clients about their children and celebrity culture.

The different discursive gender expressions of women who work at Adonis and The Executive raise the questions: What makes these women different from one another? Why do some of the women exalt masculinity and align themselves with men while the others value more conventional femininities and women's relationships? How might working for salons organized around masculinity or femininity shape the occupational choice narratives and work identities of these women? And how does such identity production symbolically reinforce or rearrange unequal relationships between women and men? After all, identities are "signs that individuals and groups use to *evoke* meaning,"[4] navigate social relations and experiences of pleasure, and claim status and power. Women who work at Adonis and The Executive show that gender identities are accomplished through everyday social processes that allow for the doing of difference,[5] whereby personal preferences and relationships of sameness and difference are produced and supported.

GENDER RELATIONSHIPS AT WORK: THE CONTEXT OF QUESTIONS AND ANSWERS

Many of the women I spoke with at The Executive discussed being held accountable by others for their decisions to work at a men's salon. When Vicky took the job working with men just two months earlier, her boyfriend said, "'Oh, yeah, you're gonna leave me for someone else, someone with more money.'" She responded: "'No. It's just something that I kind of want to do.'" Roxy told me that her friends and family ask her why she works with men and what it is like to work at a men's salon. These women work in the historically feminized beauty industry, which typically places female stylists, nail technicians, and estheticians in contact with other women.[6] Women employed at men's salons defy popular taken-for-granted assumptions about the gendered and sexualized character of their jobs. In a heteronormative culture, where people generally presume and privilege heterosexuality, few questions—popularly or scholarly—arise about the potentially sexualized character of service interactions in which women emotionally care for and physically interact with other women. We instead assume that women are drawn to this work because they are aesthetically oriented and natural caregivers, and that intimate interactions between women are devoid of sexual pleasure and tension. Both of these explanations reflect a too-narrow conception of women's interests, talents, and relationships, and essentialize women as a predictable and homogenous group. Heteronormativity, however, operates differently in relationships between women and men, so that these same jobs arouse suspicion of women in men's grooming.

When women's work defies gender norms, others struggle to make sense of them and often raise questions that make women defend not only their suitability to do the work but ultimately their gender and sexual identities.[7] What sorts of women work with men, anyway? The context in which this question arises reflects underlying assumptions about women's motivations for and experiences of working with men. First, a heteronormative culture helps to frame interactions in both salons as between women and men rather than between stylists and clients.[8] Second, the women's occupations require emotional care and physical closeness in a way many other jobs do not. This is a job that requires women and men to cross intimacy boundaries that generally constrain interactions between strangers, especially heterosocial interactions. Women are washing men's hair, rubbing their faces with exfoliate, massaging their feet, and waxing their "bikini areas." They see many of the men regularly and learn personal details about their lives. The collision of bodies and presence of physical pleasure in beauty occupations increases its association with sex work,[9] and this slippage is compounded by the salons' organizational commodification of women's heterosexual identities and conventionally feminine habitus. So, while cutting hair and clipping cuticles does not often evoke a sexual analysis by scholars[10]—although it should—when this work involves cross-gender interactions, heterosexual assumptions rise to the forefront of the women's explanations of who they are on the job.

Built into women's answers about why they work with men were expressions of just what sort of women they are, and these expressions were contextually rooted. Women at The Executive are immersed in a work culture dedicated to cultivating and celebrating masculinity. The salon is organized to produce masculine identities and includes sports television, old-style barbershop chairs, a waiting area stocked with *Golf* and *GQ* magazines, and masculinizing jargon to sell manicures as "hand-detailing" (see chapter 2). There is no room for femininity (outside of requiring hetero-feminine women workers) if owners, managers, and employees hope to convince men that the salon is a masculine place that provides clients with masculinizing services and interactions. Women who work in masculinized organizations often find they are "in a disciple environment that values masculine characteristics over feminine ones."[11] It is within a space that celebrates and privileges masculinity that the women weave narratives about their work choices and construct their sense of selves.

Women at Adonis similarly work in a salon that props-up masculinity, and which is organized around the careful cultivation of clients' masculine subjectivities. Their work experiences do not take place solely in a masculinized organization, though. Working part time at Bonita diversifies their occupational experiences and relationships, and this is reflected in their narratives about why they work at Adonis and what it is they like about their clients. While Bonita does have male clients, it is largely a women's salon. Emily, who works at both salons, told me, "Bonita is more women, like, it's like a softer, just get their hair done and relax." Workers described the salon as decorated in pinks and browns with chandeliers hanging from the ceiling. The salon serves wine instead of beer and cappuccinos and chocolates instead of Red Bull and pretzels. Patricia, who worked first at Bonita, contrasted the salon with Adonis by saying, "Bonita, it's brown. It's brown and pink, but we don't have pink inside Adonis, besides flowers. . . . The couches, they're soft and brown. . . . The glasses that your drink comes in, the cookies. It's just presented in more of a feminine way. Even the music, like, here it's loud and—we used to just have just male artists." These women are invested in two differently gendered workplaces, and their narratives were not steeped in the rejection of femininity and the exaltation of masculinity but rather in the different joys and challenges of working with both men and women.

BECOMING "MEN'S WOMEN": DISCURSIVE SAMENESS AND DIFFERENCE AT THE EXECUTIVE

Women who work in masculinized organizations confront "the dilemma of difference," in which they have to decide whether to construct themselves as "more or less different from men."[12] This is a critical dilemma since men generally hold privileged and powerful positions and projections of masculinity by men are regularly rewarded. By suggesting they are "more like men," women may try to blend in as one of the boys to reap the same benefits as celebrated men and to avoid sticking out and being defined solely as women.[13]

One of men's privileges is to symbolically represent a non-gendered location,[14] whereas women are judged as "gendered personas" rather than neutral workers.[15] Women's status is often wrapped up with their relationship to men as wives, as mothers, and as heterosexually desirable. Defining themselves as similar to men supports women's identification with dominants but also reflects their subordination to white professional-class men. This process reveals women's difficulty in attaining status on their own merits. For the white workers, this means that they serve similarly situated clients, but for the women of color, they become both racially and sexually subordinated.

Endeavoring to secure status akin to or via association with men, women at The Executive evoked "discursive separation" by highlighting distinctions in practices, traits, preferences, personalities, and social networks between themselves and other women.[16] This process of "othering" involves stereotyping women as a homogenous group and ignoring variation in women's access to privilege (along the lines of race, class, and sexuality), interests, talents, biographies, tastes, and desires.[17] These stereotypes act as "controlling images,"[18] allowing not just men but also women to objectify and degrade women as a group. By describing women as "catty," for example, women at The Executive suggest that: 1) women are not collegial; 2) men are collegial; 3) they themselves are unlike other women; and 4) therefore they are more like men and possess the positive traits of men and masculinity. These ideas construct versions of femininity that rank women and articulate unequal relationships between men and women.

Women at The Executive evoked discourses of sameness and difference, practicing gender so as to associate themselves with the privileged men in their chairs and distance themselves from structurally subordinated women. To accomplish this, they traded on misogyny, whereby they evoked sexist rhetoric and exalted narrow definitions of men and masculinity as superior to women and femininity.[19] They identified with men and with the expressions of supposed masculine behavior, but at the expense of women as a group. These narratives resist their subordinated positions in relationship to men, whom they are occupationally obligated to serve, and, at the same time, position them as naturally inclined to work in men's grooming.

A Preference for Working on Men

All except one stylist at The Executive worked full time at the salon. Many had never worked professionally with women because they were either trained as barbers or were hired by Veronica right out of cosmetology school. A few had previously worked with women but told me that they did not like it. Isabel, who had worked at the salon for three years when I met her, is the only stylist also doing women's hair. She works a couple days each week whipping brides' hair into I-do-up-do's and does makeup for bridal parties: "I love both [men and women's hair]. I do women's weddings; I do hair and makeup for weddings. I love that. I always have fun. I don't have [a] problem to work with women and I don't have [a] problem to work with guys. I love both. My boss, she says, 'Are you thinking to stop working with females? Are you gonna come with us full time?' I can't, because I love [to] work with women also. I love [to] work with them." Isabel was one of only two stylists at The Executive who admitted enjoying working on women. Nell, a new hire, was the other.

After having worked at The Executive for only a few weeks, Nell already yearned to cut women's hair. She and her brother were raised by their father, and she had worked in construction before enrolling in cosmetology school; so Nell had assumed that she would enjoy working at a men's salon. She believed that she "understood them." Evoking the same sort of discourse about knowing men as Martha, Nell had not foreseen becoming bored with men's hair. She found herself giving "just like the basic layered cut" over and over again, and she said that if The Executive drew a more diverse clientele (men from different subcultures such as punks and greasers, or perhaps men of different racial backgrounds), her work would be more variable and presumably more fun. She especially wanted to work in a rockabilly inspired salon. Women's hair, Nell said, usually allows stylists to display their "creative side," and so she was already thinking of leaving The Executive. "I will say that I did not go to school and spend X amount of dollars to do men's hair. I'm kind of at a crossroads right now . . . I like men's hair . . . [but] the artistic side is not there." Unhappy with both the lack of creativity she felt she could exercise at The Executive and the lack of tips during training, it was no surprise that Nell did not finish Veronica's eight-week training program. Citing a "poor attitude," Veronica told me that she let Nell go shortly after I had interviewed her. My conversations with Nell and Isabel revealed that there is not a lot of room at The Executive for women who do not adopt ideological frames that naturalize their choices to work on men. Veronica asks Isabel to consider leaving women's hair altogether, and Nell refused to accept the collective discourse resonating in the salon that celebrates masculinity over femininity and privileges service interactions with men.

While Isabel and Nell value and enjoy working on women's hair, they are outliers at The Executive. Most of the women essentialized sex and gender to hold men up as more preferable clients than women. "A woman's energy is more emotional," Martha claimed. Aggie elaborated on this, saying, "Women can be a lot more—I think it's like emotionally difficult to work with . . . with the women." She said that in the past, "It was always just too emotionally draining on me to deal with, to listen to people's problems all day long." Some women told me stories of having always known they wanted to work on men. June, for example, decided in cosmetology school that she wanted to work with men. Although her first job was at Sassoon, where she cut and styled mainly women's hair, her goal was to work in men's hair. "Just being in hair school, I knew right away I wanted to just do men's hair," she said. "And then after I got done with cosmetology school, I actually worked at Sassoon's, which is a pretty high-end salon, and they do more women than men. I still knew I wanted to do men's [hair]."

Although Joanne, a stylist, did not go straight into men's grooming—instead cutting children's hair for eight years before joining The Executive—she told me that her desire to work on men began in school, where she found that working with women required extensive emotional labor. "So I worked with a lot of women in school, and I have no patience for them, whatsoever. I'm not a very patient person, so it takes a lot of patience for women. . . . They require a lot more attention." "They get all mad" when they are not happy with their hair, she explained. While Joanne gives the impression that men are easygoing about their hair, clients I spoke with said they have no qualms about leaving their stylists if they were not happy with their haircuts. Dan, who likes to say he goes to The Executive for the ballgames, told me, "All I want is for the haircut to be really good. If I weren't getting that, I don't think the TV sets and the nice people would keep bringing me back." He went on: "I would sit in the back of a pickup truck once a month if I thought the haircut was better."

Stylists at The Executive did not generally seek out work at the men's salon, despite their claims they never wanted to do women's hair. Several women said that they came to work at The Executive by stumbling on Veronica's Craigslist advertisements for stylists. Veronica also recruits stylists at trade shows and when she gives hair demos at cosmetology schools. It is unclear whether her stylists would have otherwise sought employment at a men's salon. Instead, some of them saw Veronica's invitation to apply to her salon as an opportunity to gain the experience and expertise in men's hair that they did not receive in school. Nell exemplified this idea: "At our school we didn't learn much [about men's hair], so getting a formal education, formal training in how to cut a proper haircut for men was really appealing. . . . The education is great [at The Executive]." While June and Joanne suggested their preferences for men's hair and dislike of working on women preceded their employment at The Executive, other stylists appeared to have developed discourses of sameness and difference after having come to work with men. Shared rhetoric about who they are in relationship to men suggests that an informal yet preexisting and institutionalized cultural discourse circulates at the salon and informs the women's occupational choice narratives.

"The Way I Think Is More Masculine"

The Executive's motto, "We talk male, understand male!" reverberated in women's descriptions of themselves. Several women used this motto to explain why they are well suited to work in a men's salon and why clients are drawn to The Executive, suggesting men of course choose a salon in which beauty providers are similarly interested in sports, can talk about the economy, are not emotionally needy, and know how men like their hair. In this way, women not only drew similarities between themselves and men, but also distanced themselves from other women. Brinn, the receptionist who deals with jealous wives, said that clients flock to The Executive because the employees are "men's women":

KRISTEN: What else do you think the men are coming in for?

BRINN: We have amazing stylists who are extremely talented. They know what's—they're current; they're up-to-date. They know what's fashionable. They really know how to cut many different styles of hair. They really know how to connect with the men. They're men's women, you know what I mean? They're just able to really connect with them. . . .

KRISTEN: Men's women?

BRINN: Or, like, a man's woman. Somebody who's still able to be—I don't want to say "sexy" in the workplace. They still look at them like, "Wow, she's a great woman. She's able to sit here. She can talk sports with me." And they like that.

"Men's women" was a label reserved for the ultimate woman, one who can both "talk sports" and maintain her heterosexual attractiveness, and so it is an identity for men. It not only aligns women with their clients, but also situates their tastes, behaviors, and appearances as available for men's pleasure and consumption. The women insisted it was their inherent similarities to men that propelled them into men's grooming in the first place. "We are more like a man," Isabel told me.

Yet it is precisely because these women met culturally and locally valorized feminine standards and heteronormative aesthetics that they were able to comfortably construct themselves as similar to men. Not everyone can get away with this. Women athletes cross gender boundaries by bulking up or playing aggressive sports, and they often face accusations of appearing too manly or are assumed by others to be lesbians.[20] Women at The Executive do not risk losing gender or sexual status by discursively claiming a masculine disposition. This is because despite *saying* they are more like men, they end up *doing* femininity by emotionally and physically caring for clients, and by performing heterosexual aesthetic labor (see chapters 3 and 4). They constructed organizational identities as men's women from the comfortable position of gender and sexual privilege.

Like Martha, who opened this chapter, many women who work at The Executive said they tend to have few female friends, and that they get along better with men. Faith, for example, said that outside of work she rarely interacts with women and has only a couple of "girlfriends." "I guess I don't have a ton of interaction with other women other than the women that I work with and my girlfriends. I only have a couple girlfriends, so it's not like I'm surrounded by a lot of them." When I asked Faith, a stylist, if there is anything unique about working with men, she said, "I like working with men. I've always seemed to get along with men a lot better than I do with women, anyway." Not having many women friends or preferring men as friends might sound like a personal preference, but the larger pattern of women at The Executive weaving narratives about how little they like women reflects an institutionalized "repudiation of the feminine."[21] Masculinities scholar Michael Kimmel describes this repudiation as integral to male domination. Repudiating, or rejecting and degrading, women and femininity (by hurling insults, making jokes, etc.) is key to supporting hegemonic masculinity and the current gender order. This misogynistic rhetoric gives less value to practices, artifacts, and people (women and gay men) that are associated with femininity. By rejecting women as less desirable friends and clients, and by highlighting their shared interests and attitudes with a largely invariant group of men, workers at The Executive forged gender identities at the cost of women as a group.

Kendra, who had worked at The Executive for a year and a half, said that she does not see herself as particularly feminine: "I'm more of a—like, the way I think is more masculine." She explained that, "It's kind of hard for me to get along with females. I'm not really a girly-girl." Kendra did not clarify what it means to think in a "more masculine" way, but it is clear that she conflates being masculine—or more like men—with not being feminine. If being feminine is synonymous with being emotionally needy, illogical, disliking sports, and unable to talk about the economy or latest in sports news, then Kendra is cool and collected, logical, and up on the NFL draft.

In a workplace organized around the celebration of masculinity, the women who work at The Executive are able to create situationally valued identities as men's women. Faith told me that she gets along with men because, "Sometimes [I] act like a guy, too." She said, "It's definitely true, at least for me. But I've always kind of been that way. I'm girly, but I'm also a tomboy. I go play paintball, but get dressed up and go out. I'm kind of—I've always been that way. And I've always found that I got along better with guys than girls, even before I started working here." Faith allowed flexibility in her expressed gender identity, showing that practicing gender is contextual as she frames herself as a "tomboy" on the paintball field but "girly" when she dresses up for a night on the town. This tomboy rhetoric, while associating Faith with the masculinized sport paintball, is not as politically transgressive as some women suggested. This is because, as gender scholar Judith Lorber notes, "Now that previously masculine activities, such as playing basketball, have become acceptable for young girls, as has unisex clothing, the scope of cross-gender marks of differentness predicting a nonconventional adulthood for women has considerably diminished."[22] Little girls might roll around in the dirt and play football with their brothers, but this does not predict nonconforming adult gender expressions. While boys and men are still stigmatized if they play with Barbies or wear dresses, others do not necessarily see girls and women who play paintball or wear jeans as the antithesis of feminine.

Women rarely describe themselves as "tomboys" in the present sense.[23] Martha, for example, described herself as having been a tomboy as a child. "Tomboy" captures the women's behavior as young girls and helps to make sense of practices that were not gender conforming. "Tomboy" does not mean "boy," though; rather, it is a term women deploy to show their disdain for conventional definitions of, and often the constraints that come with, femininity.[24] So, while it suggests gender transgression, "tomboy" may also uphold a dichotomy of masculinity and femininity. Instead of gender being a culturally constructed continuum with multiple ways of being feminine, deploying the notion of the "tomboy" suggests that girls and women are either masculine or feminine, and ties a particular set of behaviors, tastes, and dispositions to masculinity.

"Real Bitches": Women and Misogyny

"They're just real bitches," Kendra said of women. She was describing for me the difference between working with men versus women and why she would never want to cut women's hair. "Doing women's hair, there's some women that you're just dreading when they're coming in. Ugh! Women are a pain in the ass," she said. "There's no pleasing them. They've got issues. They sit in your chair and you feel it right away. It's not a good experience." It made me uncomfortable to hear Kendra, and other women at The Executive, describe women in such a negative way. Despite us both being women, Kendra seemed quite comfortable making degrading remarks about women. Perhaps she believed such a description was a true reflection of women's sex-linked traits, or perhaps she figured I would agree with her. Either way, labeling women as "bitches" explained them away as inarguably undesirable clients and reflected the practice of misogyny associated with men and the perpetuation of sexism.

In her book *Female Chauvinist Pigs*, journalist Ariel Levy demonstrates how women buy into different cultural repertoires of misogyny that work against their interests.[25] While feelings of empowerment might wash over women as they make provocative decisions about how to display their bodies and how to represent sexuality and femininity, their behavior can also uphold long established sexist ideas about women as sexual objects whose bodies belong to men. Similarly, women employed at The Executive portrayed women in stereotypically narrow and negative ways as hard-to-please, overly emotional, pains-in-the-ass who are better off avoided.

Working at a men's salon thus becomes the logical choice for women who are looking to avoid the difficulties women supposedly create within such service work interactions.

The receptionists, stylists, and nail technicians at The Executive pointed out four things particular to women that made them "a pain in the ass" to work with. They framed women as too emotional, unrealistic, invested in "meaningless" conversations, and overall just "obnoxious." These points uphold misogyny as they indicate hatred or dislike for women as a group. Misogyny—along with homophobia, heterosexuality, and violence—is a tool often deployed by men in an effort to protect their privilege during socio-historical crises in masculinity[26] and to draw both personal and group associations with hegemonic—or rewarded definitions of— masculinity. Yet scholars overlook how, why, to what end, and in what context women wield misogyny.[27] Women might access well-established, culturally embedded, and easily accessible misogynistic rhetoric to distance themselves from other women and to align themselves with more privileged men, but it also supports a system in which women as a group have less power and value than similarly situated men.

"Women can be a lot more—I think it's like emotionally difficult to work with [them]," Bridget laughs. "You know, guys . . . With the women, it was always just too emotionally draining on me to deal with, to listen to people's problems all day long. Guys don't really want to come in here and talk about their problems so much." Bridget overlooked the fact that men indeed exercise entitlement to women's emotional labor, whereby women affirm men's thoughts and feelings. The women at Adonis and The Executive perform a lot of emotional management as they both negotiate men's potential qualms about being pampered and field men's sexual remarks, jokes, and flirtatious comments in ways that maintain men's comfort. Employers tend to hire women to do interactive service work because they see women as naturally docile and caring (i.e., feminine).[28] In salon work, women become the appropriately gendered person to provide clients with a caring touch, a friendly smile, and a sympathetic ear. While I cannot say for sure if stylists helped men work through personal problems, they certainly saw themselves as confidantes (see chapter 4).

Mirabel, who was just out of cosmetology school and currently in training at The Executive, said that when she graduated she had wanted to work with men *and* women. However, now that she was working with men, she realized, "I don't like the drama that a lot of the women bring to female salons, the attitude. It's not my thing. I'm not for attitudes, I'm not for drama." The fact that her perspective on women shifted only after beginning work at The Executive—and was not based on actual work experience with women—suggests the ideological repudiation of women as dramatic and high-maintenance clients was an existing and normalized rhetoric that circulated in the salon and provided women with available gender conceptions to help convince others of why they would do this work.

In addition to causing "drama," June described women as unrealistic about the aesthetics they can achieve through the purchase of salon services. Men, she said, know that no matter how much money they spend or how skilled their stylist, they will never look like Brad Pitt. "As far as just working with men . . . I think they have a better perception of reality. . . . I think they're not looking to look like Brad Pitt, whereas women, they think that we can perform miracles and make them look like superstars, which is kind of not really feasible." June believes that women are often disappointed that their haircuts do not dramatically improve their appearances and so are less loyal than men, willing to hop from stylist to stylist until they find the elusive perfect haircut.

Bridget added that women have unrealistic expectations because they believe they deserve perfection. "A client asked me the other day what's the difference between working with men and women. And I said to him, 'I find the difference is that women expect more than what they're paying for. Men expect the dollar amount, and they expect good service, but women expect more because they think they're worth more.'" While speaking more generally about men and women, Bridget assures her client that working with men is preferable because they are more reasonable than women. Loretta, who was sitting-in on our conversation, agreed: "I think there's a kind of aura of entitlement [with women]."

While men are generally expected to be assertive and demanding, and to know what they want, women who express the same attitudes are popularly framed as problems. Others might label them as "bitches," denouncing them as too sure, domineering, and aggressive—meaning too masculine.[29] Describing women as unrealistic or entitled does the same thing: it controls women's behavior so they do not express discontent but instead evoke a silence that maintains women as feminine, docile, and agreeable. Further, the idea that women are uppity and think they are "worth more" suggests they do not have the same entitlement, privilege, or value as men, whom others are more likely to interpret as appropriately masculine for being decisive and for demanding they get the product they feel they paid for. This is particularly poignant since women make less money than men on average.[30] They spend more money on beauty services and products than men but are not supposed to expect their hard-earned dollar to procure excellent service. So, although women who work at The Executive argue that men complain less often about their haircut, this is often not substantiated by their personal experiences and does not mean men are more realistic or satisfied with their haircuts than women. Not only did men tell me they would find a new stylist if they were ever unhappy with their haircut, but stylists also mentioned men bringing in photos of celebrities for inspiration.

Stylists and nail technicians at The Executive told me that they work at a men's salon partly because they do not like talking with women. Joanne, who had worked at The Executive for almost eleven years, said, "I love [working with men]." She went on to explain, "It's obviously different than working with women. I didn't want to work with women. . . . I just like talking to men all day long. I'd rather talk to men all day than with women!" Most of the women said they prefer talking with men; since their jobs require constant talking, this is an important aspect of their job satisfaction. Women like to talk about their families and kids, they said, and they find these topics boring. "I'm sorry, but it bores me to death," Bridget said. "I love my kids, but I don't put 'em on this pedestal and bore everyone else to death about how wonderful they are." When she is at work, she would rather talk about other things: "Yeah, I prefer to talk about things like what's going on in the news, what's going on in the economy, rather than talking about—I mean, I have kids and I love my kids, but I don't want to listen to someone talk about their kids' achievements."

Aggie insinuated women have aimless conversations. "Maybe it's part of the reason why [working with men] works better for me, you know, because it's hard for me to just have, like, meaningless conversation. Guys, if they don't want to talk, they're not gonna talk, and if they're gonna say something, it's usually a little bit more for a reason." The women associated uninteresting or unimportant topics of conversations with women, and suggested men talk about more elevated and engaging topics. The disdain workers held for mommy talk allowed them to separate themselves from women with mere domestic lives, reflecting the "mommy wars" that discursively separate working mothers from stay-at-home mothers and reduce women to their roles as wives and mothers.[31] Stylists who groom other women might indeed find that they talk with clients about family life, since class, occupation, race, and sexual orientation might separate them, and thus family is something they have in common. Of course, recognizing their shared experiences with other women as mothers undermines women's discursive separation from femininity and feminized familial roles and ignores the fact that men might indeed want to—and sometimes do—talk about their families with their stylists and nail technicians.[32]

Even the receptionists at The Executive said they prefer working with men, claiming men are less "obnoxious" than women. Brinn and Julie, both young receptionists, do not interact with clients as closely or intimately as the stylists and nail technicians, but they are the first and often last person the men see at the salon. They greet men, fetch them beer, cash them out, book their next appointments, and follow-up with them to make sure they were satisfied with their haircuts, manicures, and manscaping services. Seeing the irony in being a woman herself, Brinn was hesitant to negatively stereotype women. "Honestly, and I don't even want to say this, because I *am* a woman, but guys are so much more laid-back than women." She imagines women would hold grudges against her, or "harp" on her, for innocent mistakes like scheduling errors:

> I feel like even if I provided the same type of customer service at a women's salon, if there was a scheduling error, instead of a man just being like, "I understand," if we did make an error and I was to call them and say, "I'm so sorry, we made a scheduling error, here's what I can offer you, if this will work for you. If not, let's work on it." Obviously, [men are] gonna be a little upset, but they're always like, "Ok, you know what? No problem. Things happen. Thank you. You've always been on top of things. I can do this." And it's over with. I feel like a woman would be more inclined to hold a grudge, continue to harp on it, want to go to management, just be obnoxious.

Although Brinn's salon work experience is limited to The Executive, she expressed certainty that working in a women's salon would mean dealing with fickle clients. Julie, a college student who worked part time at the salon, also assumed that working with men makes her life "easy" because "women aren't laid-back" whereas men "don't expect too much."

Working Alongside—Not On—Women

"I really like the ladies I work with," Aggie told me. Outside of work, she spends time with Martha, June, and Kendra; they catch movies together and go out for drinks and appetizers. "I think they're all great," she said. "And when we all get together, it's fun." Declarations of affection for the women they worked with peppered the occupational narratives of employees at The Executive. They created close friendships with the other stylists, nail technicians, and receptionists whom they see almost every day. This declaration contradicts both their claims to gravitate to men for friendships and their misogynist attitudes about women as exhausting and emotional. I was curious as to how these women could reinforce degrading stereotypes about women while also rooting their job satisfaction partly in the pleasurable relationships they develop with female coworkers.

The contradiction between not wanting to work *on* women and enjoying working *alongside* women did not pose an ideological dilemma for women employed at The Executive. They were able to form close bonds with the women they worked with because they saw them as similarly exceptional men's women. This was no coincidence, Martha suggested, telling me that Veronica, the owner, sifts out typical "catty" women during the hiring process, and that this is why "all of us girls get along." She explained that Veronica completes "extensive interviewing" with potential hires to make sure she does not bring someone into the fold who "doesn't fit" and hires only women who are "very open and friendly." Martha was sure that hiring was organizationally orchestrated so as to create a team of "easy-going" women, and thus to make the men's salon a uniquely gendered environment.

The women characterized typical salons as female-dominated places rife with drama. Drawing from her previous work experiences, June described many salons as fostering environments in which women form exclusionary relationships. "I've worked at salons where it's very cliquey and it's almost like a sorority, and it's not fun." The Executive, she said, does not fall into this trope because it caters to a male clientele; men, she claimed, do not form alliances and cliques. Feeding into the specter of homosociality, June suggested the salon was a men-only place: "Since we don't have women in the salon, we don't really have to worry about offending anybody, for the most part." June believed that by working in a men's salon she avoids both easily offended female clients and otherwise "cliquey" female coworkers. Women who work at The Executive do not see the salon as female dominated, despite the fact that women workers often outnumber male clients, especially on weekdays when business is slow. They do not count themselves as typical women because they see themselves as "more like men." This upholds The Executive as a place for men and for women who are like men, or who see themselves as honorary men. The women expressed a collective gender identity around *not* counting as women, and thus it made sense they could build and express friendships with each other.

Women who work at The Executive claimed men help to "balance" the "estrogen" in salons. They argued that too many women in one place is a recipe for disaster. Nell, who was raised by her dad, was adamant that when "you're stuck in a room with thirty girls for X amount of hours a week," it creates tension between workers on the shop floor. Recalling her experiences in cosmetology school where she spent most of her time with women, she said, "I think that no-drop-of-testosterone kind of environment, it just breeds craziness." Aggie agreed that men help to placate the "tizzy" women create when left on their own: "Part of the reason why I like the girls here, we're relaxed and cool, is because we're working on guys." Men, she suggested, make women better people by taming their natural propensity to get "carried away": "That balances it out. In women's hair salon[s] I worked in, every one I worked in, it was just kind of like catty. There's too much estrogen. [Laughs] Women get all carried away and in a tizzy. Here, it's like—I think the balance of the testosterone and our relationship[s] with each other, too, between the girls and the clients, just kind of makes it a bit more harmonious. [Laughs] Balanced." Despite the fact that men and women have both (and often fluctuating levels of) estrogen and testosterone,[33] Nell recalled long-held beliefs about the link between sex, hormones, and behavior. The idea that women are controlled by their hormones and are naturally more emotional than men has roots in nineteenth-century medical explanations of "female hysteria."[34] Hysteria was used as a diagnosis that naturalized women as weaker and as less capable, predictable, and rational than men.[35] This androcentric rationalization reduced women to their biology and supported (and continues to support) both the exclusion of women from public roles and the privileging of men as more rightly represented in decision-making positions and high-status occupations.

In case there is any suspicion that women employed at The Executive threaten the calm energy of the salon with their rampant estrogen, they suggested that clients' testosterone is a great equalizer. Too much estrogen (i.e. women), they suggested, is undesirable and will create tense relationships in the workplace. What is desirable and helpful is the presence of men. This reinforces the idea that men and women are complementary opposites.[36] The presence of testosterone (men) is supposed to equalize the otherwise hysteric behavior that will surely escalate in female-dominated spaces, where women's behavior is reduced to their reproductive biology. Testaments to the positive effects of testosterone are significant because it ranks men and women according to sexist presumptions about the operations of hormones.

VALUING WOMEN'S CULTURE: ADONIS

Women employed at Adonis work in a masculinized space that is organized similarly to The Executive. Tyler, the owner, created a space that is supposed to appeal to men in its sleek décor, beer, Xbox game systems, privatizing layout, and titillating commercials. And so I was surprised the women did not discursively practice gender like those at The Executive. When women working at Adonis explained how they arrived at the salon, they highlighted their accidental employment at Adonis, their part-time status in men's grooming, and their ongoing investment in doing women's hair and nails. Unlike workers at The Executive, almost all of the women at Adonis split their time between the masculinized men's salon and the more feminized women's salon, Bonita, with its glass chandeliers and feminine color scheme. Investing in two differently gendered workplaces, women at Adonis did not describe suspicious family and friends who wanted to know why and how they work so closely with men. Vacillating between workplaces, the women did not stake a clear interest in the discursive reproduction of masculine privilege and their own status.

Women at Adonis did not face the same dilemma of difference and were not as preoccupied with being one of the boys as those at The Executive. While they were certainly integral to Adonis's goals of producing a feeling of class-privileged masculinity, the women did not draw on these informal job requirements to carve out occupational choice narratives and workplace gender identities as "more like men." Going back-and-forth between salons, the women were required and encouraged to display gender differently at the two places, and both management and client expectations differed, as did the actual work processes. There were moments when some of the beauty workers made it clear that they enjoyed engaging in feminine consumer cultural and bodily practices and interacting with other women. While the women's narratives sometimes conflated sex and gender, they also carved out a more egalitarian relationship between men and women, masculinity and femininity.

Instead of suggesting there is something unique about them as "men's women" that attracted them to men's grooming, they wove stories that recognized benefits to working with men while also valuing women as clients and femininity as an enjoyable set of bodily repertoires and work processes. Invested in two differently gendered salons, where masculinity or femininity are reproduced and highly valued as processes linked to clients' pleasure and the bottom line, the women develop a more flexible narrative about gender and who they are, or who they can be, at work. They approach gender in a more flexible manner and have more diversified gendered work experiences that inform their narratives about their work experiences, opportunities, and identities.

Stumbling into Men's Grooming

Mary came to work at Adonis quite accidently and had no intention of working in men's grooming. Commuting long distances to her previous workplace, she wanted to find a job that was closer to her parents, with whom she was living. She knew that Bonita's neighborhood was filled with "a lot of wealthy men and women," and so she could presumably carve out a lucrative living there. She also believed working in the area could be enjoyable because the locals are "so down-to-earth, so laid back, so just accepting and really cool." In her hunt for a new job that filled her requirements of "good people, good salon, good products," Mary compiled a "listing of all the different salons" in the area, and went door-to-door with her résumé. She "first walked into Bonita" looking for work: "I dropped by Bonita, and [a woman] said, 'Actually the owner of the spa is mostly over at Adonis. You should drive by Adonis.'"

While Mary had heard of Adonis, it was not on her list of salons to apply to, and she was surprised that Tyler and his wife owned both Adonis and Bonita. "I didn't know it was the same owners. So, I was like, 'OK, I'll go by there.'" Tyler was not at the salon when she stopped by, so she left her résumé at the front desk and received a call from him later that evening. "He totally called that night and we met a couple days later and I started." Mary was unsure about working in men's hair and did not initially think she would like Adonis because she prefers to cut and style women's hair. But the job was located in the middle of town, provided her the opportunity to wait for a position to become available at Bonita, and, importantly, the job was hers if she wanted it. Tyler eventually did offer Mary a part-time gig at Bonita, in addition to Adonis. When I interviewed her, she estimated that 70 percent of her time is spent shoring up men's hair and said that she does women's hair one or two days each week.

Stories like Mary's gave me the impression that Adonis has a difficult time hiring and retaining stylists precisely because it focuses on men. The salon is stocked full of good-looking women largely because Tyler's wife, who runs Bonita, refers them. Veronica did not have waves of women seeking positions at The Executive, either; she works hard to recruit stylists. The women at both Adonis and The Executive were steeped in a work culture that elevated men and privileged masculinity, but those at Adonis did not collectively develop and project masculinized identities around the rejection of women and the privileging of men as superior people and clients. Like Mary, they carved out occupational choice narratives that reflected their desires to do women's hair and accidental introduction into men's grooming.

While Ryan and Joshua cut hair only at Adonis, many of the women working at Adonis spend time at Bonita. Patricia and Elsie, for example, do hair at Adonis once a week to accommodate male clients they used to see at Bonita. "A lot of my [male] clients at Bonita came over here," Elsie told me. She explained that when Adonis opened, much of her male clientele said they would feel more comfortable in a men's salon, and so Adonis hired her part time to retain the men she had formed relationships with at Bonita. "I think some guys that went over [to Bonita] are more used to being over there, until they try Adonis," she said. The geographical closeness of Adonis and Bonita, which are only about two miles from each other, as well as the salons' shared ownership, makes it possible for women to move seamlessly between them to better serve and retain their male clients. If Elsie did not also cut hair at Adonis, she would run the risk of losing regular clients who are intrigued by or more comfortable in a men's salon. Some of her clients are more loyal to her than to the salon, she said, and are willing to schedule an appointment at Bonita if they cannot get in with her at Adonis. But these men prefer Adonis and would miss the free mini-facial that accompanies their haircut if they ever left. She explained: "So when they come over to Bonita, because I'm not at Adonis every day, they're like, 'Oh, I miss the facial, bummer, I wish I could have had that.' So they really do like all those little things that we do for them over here."

Some women who work at Adonis are biding their time while they wait for a position to open up at Bonita. Holly, a twenty-two-year-old stylist, told me that she does not want to work with men, and that although she had been at Adonis for over a year she was holding out hope that she would be transferred to Bonita fulltime. Similar to Mary, Holly had originally applied to Bonita. "I actually applied to Bonita," she said, because "I never specialized in men's hair ever in my life. But Tyler—actually [his wife], told me to come over here and look and see the salon. So, I came by the same day, I dropped off my résumé, and then I don't know. Tyler was there, and he just hired me right off the—he was like, 'Why don't you work here? Would you be interested in working with men?' And I was like, 'I guess, yeah, whatever.'" Holly "fell into" men's hair but is still "really stuck on" Bonita because she "really wanted to work there."

In contrast to stylists and nail technicians at The Executive, Holly and other women working at Adonis explained that they were not experts in men's grooming. First, they agreed that men's hair is not a topic covered extensively by cosmetology instructors and that they had to learn how to cut and style men's hair "on the job." Second, they aren't men. After a year of working at Adonis, Holly still does not think of herself as an expert in men's hair because, "Well, I'm not a dude," she said. "Technically I don't really wear my hair very short, and so . . . I get frustrated because I wish they knew what they wanted." Unlike women working at The Executive, Holly did not claim that she talks like and understands men. Instead, she suggested that as a woman who has long hair, she cannot fully know what her clients want in a haircut unless they tell her. Practicing gender by linking herself with women and distancing herself from men, Holly highlighted her identity as a woman and made space for a flexible occupational choice narrative that explains her interest in both men's and women's grooming.

Jesse is the only woman at Adonis who works full time with men. She enjoys cutting women's hair, but will get her "fix" by doing her friends' and family members' hair. She also occasionally cuts women's hair at Bonita, if a friend or an old client requests her. Jesse explained that she chose to focus on men's hair because she believes there is more money in it. As a single mother of two, she explained, "Initially, I went to Adonis full time because I made a lot more money there and I was just busier and it comes down to raising two kids by myself, so it was kind of like, wherever I'm making a little better money and busier." While a stylist working at Bonita might see twenty clients in a week, Jesse sees an average of twelve to eighteen men each day at Adonis. Mary, who works with Jesse, was also thinking of moving to men's grooming full time: "With a woman, you're having to apply the color, wait, take it out, shampoo their hair, cut their hair, style, blow dry." She points out that it takes longer to do women's hair, which might require multiple lengthy processes. Men, on the other hand, are quicker to turn over. Other women, however, argued that there is more money in women's hair because extensions, coloring, and straightening cost more than men's simple cuts, and because they can juggle multiple clients at once (cutting one woman's hair while another's hair sets under the dryer).

Differently Gendered Experiences: "Guy Mode" versus Corporeal Artist

Men and women's salons are "two different worlds," workers at Adonis told me. They see Adonis and Bonita as distinct from one another in terms of décor, vibe, type of clients, and the sort of worker they are at the different salons. They described Adonis as "laid back" and "casual," and they painted Bonita as a feminized and high-end space with wine instead of beer. Patricia, who splits her time between the two salons, said that she dresses and acts differently at Adonis and Bonita. At Bonita, she is more likely to wear "heels or a dress and I might wear more jewelry and do my hair differently." The workers see men and women as essentially different and thus appropriately divided between salons—with men in the sleek yet beer-serving Adonis and women in the fancy cappuccino-brewing Bonita.

While a male clientele offers stylists fast money and casual revolving interactions, working with women allows them to express their creativity and bond with other women over conversations about beauty culture. Similar to The Executive, women at Adonis work in a place organized around the privileging of masculinity, but their diversified work experiences that split them between men's and women's salons inform their opinions about men and women as "different creatures," yet similarly enjoyable. This discursive typification of men and women allows workers to raise up women and femininity as worthy of appreciation and sources of both creative workplace identities and enjoyable work experiences—although this comes with its own set of problems.

Working on Men. Most of the women came to work at Adonis quite accidentally, and although many still have their eye on a career working in women's hair, they do enjoy working in what they referred to as a "laid-back" atmosphere with men who are "fun." Gabrielle, for example, likes that she can "let loose" in the salon, bantering back-and-forth with the men and making jokes. You can slip into "guy mode" when interacting with men, Jackie said. When I asked her to define what exactly "guy mode" is, she explained, "Guy mode, yeah, like, 'Hey, what's up? What's goin' on? How are you?' That's guy mode . . . men are more casual. It's, 'Hey, how are you?'"

Peppered with televisions and video game consoles, Adonis sometimes reminded me more of an upscale arcade than a hair salon. These sorts of amenities mark the salon as a masculine space and encourage rowdy behavior as men cheer on their favorite football teams or establish high scores on Grand Theft Auto. Bonita does not have televisions, and so interactions in the salon are more focused on intimate conversations between clients and stylists. The stylists identified the gendered differences between Adonis and Bonita in terms of décor, amenities, and interactions with clients, but they rarely connected these things. Talking with men about sports, for example, makes sense when clients are watching sports TV while having their haircut, and a casual environment marked by beer and free pizza Wednesdays sets the stage for relaxed interactions between clients and stylists. The glass chandelier, heart-shaped chocolates, and champagne glasses at Bonita, on the other hand, symbolize not only a high-end space for women but also create a more formal atmosphere in which workers feel they need to dress up. In this way, the differently gendered salons enable and constrain behavior, interactions, embodiments, and ultimately workers' understanding of and appreciation for these workplaces.

Like employees at The Executive, women working at Adonis said that they enjoy interacting with men because they are "easy to deal with." They described men as pliable clients who yield beauty expertise to women and often know little about the intricacies of hair mousse and paraffin pedicures.

Jackie elaborated on this, telling me that women tend to be more educated in beauty culture and repertoires than men, and are thus "trend spotters." From an early age, many women are initiated via their mothers, sisters, and female friends into beauty culture, and they have long consumed and cultivated staunch ideas about products and styles.[37] As a result, workers suggested that women more often expect to forge a grooming plan in collaboration with their stylists, nail technicians, or esthetician, participating as co-experts.[38] Whereas women are in search of a particular "look," they told me that men "just come in and say, 'I want you to tell me what I need and send me on my way.'" "I like working with women," Jackie said, "but men I find much easier than women." She especially finds it easier to sell men products. Men are increasingly educated consumers who pay attention to their appearances and what they slather on their bodies or in their hair; yet, they defer to women as beauty experts.

One stylist described herself as slipping into "guy mode" when she talks with her Adonis clients. If men are easy to get along with, collegial, and unemotional about things, then being a "guy" means engaging in a relaxed way. In an occupation that requires workers to talk with clients all day long, it is not a surprise they might enjoy light conversation that requires less energy and less emotional labor. It is easy to start a dialogue with men, stylists said. They ask men, "Did you watch the Lakers game last night? What'd you do this weekend?" At the same time, while they held up this as enjoyable and a product of working with men rather than in a masculinizing place, they did not characterize guy mode as preferable to their experiences with women at Bonita. And the quick turnover of clients means that while working at Adonis is fast paced, they did not have to hold long, ongoing conversations with clients like they do at Bonita, where women might spend two to three hours for one appointment.

Slipping into guy mode does not mean the women see themselves as "men's women" at work. Unlike the stylists, nail technicians, and receptionists at The Executive, women at Adonis not once described themselves as "more like men" or as "tomboys." They also did not suggest that they preferred interacting with men. Instead, these workers highlighted the fluidity and performativity of gender, whereby gender is not inherent but something created as people follow different rules or available scripts in different situations with different expectations and different people. At the same time the women revealed that guy mode is a temporal and contextual state that they move in and out of, they also associated the appropriateness of this sort of behavior with men's supposed inherent relaxed attitudes and interests in sports. Doing so, the women uphold the masculinity built into the brand image of Adonis and fulfill the salon's experiential promises to consumers. But the women also get something out of the salon's cultivation and support for "masculine" behavior and "masculine" interactions: job satisfaction and the ability to deploy and enjoy gender variability and thus less androcentric identities and gender discourses.

Working on Women. Working with men gives stylists relief from the long appointments and conversations that take place at Bonita, but many of them also said that working on women provides them something they cannot get at Adonis: a sense of creativity and artistry. Like Nell, who was unhappy giving essentially the same haircut to every client at The Executive, Patricia said that working solely at Adonis would limit her creativity. "With men," she said, "their hair's so short, it's really hard to get creative. They just sit in that same box." Cutting men's hair is quicker than women's and very routine, she explained: "It's consultation, shampoo, haircut, rinse out, and then at Adonis we do the hot towel treatment, come back, style 'em, clean up, and next person. So it's very—it's kind of like a machine, I guess. It's the same thing. Most of my clients, since they're repetitive, they don't do a lot of change." So, while Adonis sells men on a pampered experience, it is also a methodical service that embeds workers in a cycle of predictable workdays and heavy client turnover. The women workers described men as desiring "consistency" and "predictability" in their haircuts, rather than taking the time to play with different styles. Men, they said, also need to feel like they are getting their "money's worth," but do not want to be at the salon for too long. On average, stylists try to wrap up men's haircuts within thirty minutes.

Working at Bonita allows the stylists to flex their creative muscles and provides them with variability in their work. Women tend to have longer hair, use more coloring products, and are more open to experimenting with their appearances than men. Stylists indicated that this makes the work enjoyable and an important process for carving out creative identities. These women see cutting and arranging hair as a creative outlet and themselves as creative people. Their job satisfaction is greatly promoted by their ability to feel both creative and like they are honoring their motivations for entering cosmetology in the first place. Even Jesse, who decided to leave women's hair to work at Adonis full time, admitted, "I like working with women, too, and just doing women's hair, it's more to work on. More styles, the styling aspect, the coloring aspect. All that kind of stuff you don't really do too often with men. You do a little color with men, but that's it." While the salon offers men the same services as many women's salons, like hair coloring, Jesse said the techniques involved in these processes are quite different for men and women. Coloring at Adonis is a quick twenty-minute process, involving easily applied Redken's Color Camo to cover graying roots. Women, on the other hand, might desire layers of color and change their hair color frequently to accomplish different looks. Coloring women's hair builds autonomy and decision making into the stylists' jobs, so that they are less "mechanical." Highlighting women's hair with blonds and reds, for example, requires stylists to exercise their expertise in coloring: making decisions about what shades look best on a client and assessing where to place color so as to best frame a client's face or create a dramatic effect.

Women's hair is a reprieve from the quick and heavily routinized work at Adonis. Patricia and Elsie told me that they would "never" leave women's hair. Elsie admitted that she prefers to do men's hair, but that the autonomy and variability in doing women's hair keeps her working part time at Bonita. "There's so many different women's haircuts," Elsie said. "From short to middle length to long to extensions, I do extensions. There's so much more." Emily, a young stylist, agreed that women's hair allows her to be "a bit more creative," and that she can't imagine doing men's hair full time. "If I only did men's hair, I might commit suicide or something." Appreciating the different occupational benefits at both salons, Emily likes to move between Adonis and Bonita: "I couldn't only do men's hair . . . I like the balance of doing both. I like them both."

In addition to seeing themselves as creatively uninhibited at Bonita, stylists working with women also said they enjoy talking with women about "makeup, perfumes, and purses and vacations, family, and kids." Deploying discursive sameness, these stylists explained that they share these interests with their female clients and are similarly plugged in to a women's consumer culture and have their own family responsibilities. Instead of repudiating femininity to become extraordinary women, these stylists set themselves up as like other women and thus end up valuing women's relationships with one another as well as the shared expressions of femininity and familial experiences as wives, girlfriends, and mothers. This feeling of affinity with other women reflects the role beauty culture has long played in bringing women together, whereby they have shared skin and hair elixir recipes and created supportive communities that helped with childcare and worked politically to challenge racial oppression.[39]

At the same time, by highlighting those experiences they might share with other women, the stylists ignored differences in race, ethnicity, class, and sexuality that might separate them from their female clients. They suggested that as women they have the gender capital or cultural knowledge necessary to relate easily with women during two- to three-hour appointments. Eva, who had worked at Adonis for two and a half years, said that she enjoys the conversation she has with her female clients "'Cause women, it's easy, because you instantly relate to women." "Guys," on the other hand, "you don't instantly relate to because you're not interested in the same thing." She went on to mention Tyler's informal rule requiring stylists to keep up with current sports news in order to make men more comfortable talking about "manly" things at Adonis. "Some guys you try to learn to talk about things that they like [such as sports]." She finds this extra work to be boring, and prefers the more organic conversations that emerge when she speaks with female clients at Bonita. In this way, she reified gender stereotypes that assume women as a group can be characterized by their consumer practices and family roles. Room for differences that divide women, break with stereotypes, and otherwise challenge gender dichotomies disappears in these occupational choice narratives.

Steeped in two differently gendered workplaces, stylists at Adonis wove stories about the pains and pleasures of working on men and women without privileging one over the other. At times, however, the women conflated sex and gender: stereotyping men as having narrow interests in sports and generalizing women as an inherently monolithic group with shared life experiences. After all, men too have families and are immersed in consumption, and they might even want to discuss these things with their stylists.[40] The women at Adonis suggest there is something about being a woman that bridges all other divides and connects them easily to other women. This solidifies their identities as women and creates a sense of sameness with female clients who might be more racially or financially privileged than they are.[41] The occupational choice narratives of these women reinforce gender dichotomies by discursively setting up men and women as diametrically natural opposites, but also make room to value and enjoy femininity and other women.

CONCLUSION

Scholars suggest that women can have unequal relationships but cannot subordinate one another along the lines of gender,[42] and that femininities cannot be used to oppress each other.[43] That is, race, class, and sexuality intersect with gender so that black women have less access to structural power and privilege than white women, but both occupy subordinate locations in the gender hierarchy. White women have racial privilege over black women, not gender privilege. By trading on misogyny, however, female beauty workers at The Executive show women can and do evoke discourses that together reinforce men's dominance and subordinate supposed "typical" women (or "real bitches") to extraordinary, masculinized women. They develop multiple, hierarchical femininities that are not tied to race, for example, so much as they are tied to gender, and to masculinity more specifically. Masculinity is an accessible tool by which they accomplish hierarchical rankings of women according to supposed proximities to femininities and masculinities and so bring into question what pariah femininities,[44] whereby women refuse to endorse hegemonic masculinity, might look like.

Instead of reflecting some kind of deep-seated masculine disposition, the occupational choice narratives of women at The Executive reveal that even women can "move through and produce masculinity by engaging in masculine practices."[45] They create room to imagine women who practice or embody masculinity—destabilizing the link between sex and gender—but they also reify conventional femininity as something that is both inherently characteristic and undesirable of most women. Forging identities as "one of the boys" emerges within and from a culture that celebrates men and privileges masculinity.[46] Yet women invested in various gendered workplaces "do difference" differently.[47] Women working at Adonis and Bonita weave narratives that essentialize masculinity and femininity as sex-linked, but they do so in a way that does not reproduce hierarchical relationships between them. They do not organize women according to femininities so much as they value how the differently gendered salons allow them both variability in their relationships with clients and less oppressive frames by which they make sense of their work and who they are at work. These discourses and identities are threats to masculinity as superior to femininity, and thus to male dominance.

CONCLUSION

Voted "the world's top MAG—or Man Aging Gracefully," George Clooney is publicly praised for "looking happy in his skin," "embrac[ing] middle age," and being "sexy as a brooding silver fox."[1] Depicted as effortlessly dapper, Clooney's gray hair is proof that he doesn't concern himself too much with the effects of aging; wouldn't he dye his hair if he did? All top ten MAGs, however, have full heads of hair: Brad Pitt, Johnny Depp, Daniel Craig, Matthew McConaughey, Will Smith, and so on. Not only does balding age a man, but a lack of hair has been associated historically with little civil confidence in men's leadership abilities and reputability as white-collar workers.[2] Hair acts as a symbol of virility, with Clooney's natural color separating him from men who hang desperately onto youth. At the same time though, it is no secret that Matthew McConaughey went from a receding hairline to a full head of hair, with journalists wondering if he had a hair transplant,[3] and a celebrity report claims that George Clooney travels with his own personal hairstylist, who is on hand to shore up his locks no matter where he is in the world.[4]

While popular rhetoric vacillates between veiling and revealing men's investments in aesthetic enhancement, it is clear that looking good does not have to be emasculating. For the right kind of man and under the right set of circumstances, men can and do devote a great deal of time, money, energy, and selfhood to the beauty industry without risking their associations with valorized definitions of manhood. A framework of naturalness surrounds the MAG awards, which preserves the idea that the corporeality of these high-status celebrities is distinctly masculine. Women care about how they look, men just happen to look good. The men's salons I examine in this book do something similar: they produce gendered beauty rhetoric, spaces, and experiences that can be folded into the status-enhancing narratives and experiences of class-privileged corporate men. But these men do not just deploy heterosexual and professional identities to justify their ventures into the beauty industry,[5] structures of class, sexuality, and race also shape the philosophies, marketing strategies, and labor of Adonis and The Executive.

Early on, my research was motivated by one question: What makes a men's salon a *men's* salon? Studying Adonis and The Executive was a way for me to begin understanding the larger phenomenon of men's growing consumer participation in the beauty industry. A free market supports corporations' interests rather than those of workers' and consumers'. Corporations are in constant conflict and competition to grow their power and influence in the marketplace, and one way they do this is through innovation by creating new concepts, or "formats," including men's salons and men's exfoliate. Following the cycle of the market, we see that the "conflict between existing and new formats is the driving force behind changes in the retail sector."[6] These changes take the form of new life stages and lifestyles, like "tweens" and "metrosexuals," which are accomplished through the everyday consumption of particular products and services. Looking in real time at how people relate to market innovation moves us beyond a perspective concerned solely with the bottom line.

A cultural analysis of advertisements and men's products offers rich insight into the commercial cultivation of masculinities, but I was interested in how both the organizations and the people with whom men come into contact as they pursue more beautiful bodies help to create a market-driven masculinizing endeavor. Adonis and The Executive are part of a larger industry invested in supporting and capitalizing on men's embodied identities and on cultural associations between bodies and symbolic status. The body is not separate from culture; it is shaped from a "stock of cultural skills and techniques"[7] that separates and aligns people by group membership and social mores. How we make bodies teaches us something about social relationships and power; and bodies are made in multiple ways: not only through the private application of wrinkle cream, but also through public experiences with and the cultivation of narratives around beauty. Men might get stylish haircuts at the salons, but it is in the way their stylists talk about hair and how men experience the process of getting their hair cut that supports their psychological and socially significant identities as straight, class-privileged white men. I therefore asked: How do men feel in the salons? How do they engage available amenities (do they drink beer and watch television while having their nails buffed)? What sorts of relationships do they form with the women who are charged with grooming them? These questions emerged in the field and helped me understand the multilevel social processes involved in creating men's salons. Looking at the feelings, practices, and interactions produced at Adonis and The Executive, my goals for this book have been to interrogate the popular idea that men's consumer participation in beauty is feminizing and equalizes the gender order, and to shine light on how men's commercial grooming sorts women by sexual identities and relies on gendered labor.

WHAT'S NEW?

Men have long fashioned their bodies to express, establish, and transcend their social locations, and to resist social subordination. As Michel Foucault notes, there is a "materiality of power operating on the very bodies of individuals" so that bodies carries with them the mark of social distinction,[8] whereby professional white men look different from the Mexican immigrant shoe shiner who spiffs up their loafers. While Foucault emphasizes the body as a public spectacle, I stress that meaning rests not just in the presentation of the body but also in the social exchanges that make the body.

Coming back to the example of my father, who purchased English Leather cologne at the drugstore, it is clear that his bodily maintenance was an attempt to meet the white middle-class norms of the time. Although he lacked access to the plethora of "for men" products and services that exist today, his masculinity was still linked to his (lack of) consumer habits. He escaped the outright purchase of grooming products and instead dipped into my mom's moisturizer and hair dye in the privacy of their home. Today, however, a web of manufacturers, marketers, retailers, and popular media experts support men's beauty consumption by mediating cultural associations of beauty and gender. And the value of goods and services does not come from their function so much as from their localized implications and broader meanings.[9] Hair dye, for example, darkens men's hair so they appear younger and perhaps more competent in their workplaces, but it also helps professional men to approach white-collar work expectations more generally. Men don't individually decide that it is a good idea to dye their graying roots; rather, they engage cultural practices that are symbolically significant in a particular place and at a particular time in history. They understand, even if subliminally, that they are supposed to present themselves to the world in a particular way, given who they are, and that—for especially white well-to-do men—they may be interpersonally and structurally rewarded if they meet these expectations.

The social value of beauty goods and services for men lies in the avenues by which they access them. I move beyond the meanings reflected on the surfaces of men's bodies and in the packaging of face scrub to show that the social consequences of consumerism arise as men engage with growing corporate marketing strategies, cross the threshold into new masculinized corporate spaces like Adonis and The Executive, and engage a new niche of service workers responsible for supporting their identities. These examples highlight the epistemological significance of studying actions and interactions when studying consumerism, and for studying consumerism through the lens of work. Men's public engagement with the beauty industry is a growing phenomenon, and it is this public character that simultaneously threatens men's associations with rewarded definitions of masculinity and mitigates this threat by having others bear witness to their corporeal investment. Men who are purchasing manicures at Adonis might be stored away in a back room, but they are also sitting among other well-to-do men as they wait for their appointments. Furthermore, their physical and emotional interactions with straight and conventionally gendered workers allow them to demonstrate heterosexuality for anyone who might be watching, for an imagined other, and for themselves.

A LITTLE OFF THE BACK

Marketing research discusses the importance of rebranding and reshelving beauty products so that men don't run screaming when corporations try to sell them moisturizer or styling wax.[10] These reports encourage corporations to masculinize beauty by making services and products appear different from those that women buy and apply. The rise of grooming product sales clearly exhibits the purchasing power of men, and men are heading into previously off-limit spaces, like the historically feminized hair salon, to purchase beauty services. Reshelving beauty for men goes beyond creating a "Man Zone" at H-E-B grocery stores.[11] The men's salons in this book epitomize commercial reshelving efforts, where an entire corporate space—not just an aisle—is dedicated to men's corporeal pursuits. The historically feminized hair salon is separated from women through a process of repackaging and recoding. Conventional beliefs about class, masculinity, and, less explicitly, race, organize Adonis and The Executive in ways to create a consumer experience for men who identify with the salons' spaces, amenities, and services. And it is women beauty workers who bear the brunt of mediating the cultural significance of these things for men.

The men's grooming industry is built on the backs of women beauty workers, with the worker-client relationship critical in creating a willing male beauty consumer. By looking at how these relationships operate on the ground, this book reveals the dynamics of a service industry that recodes the meaning of beauty by drawing from and reproducing gender inequalities. A largely female workforce of hair stylists, barbers, nail technicians, estheticians, and even salon receptionists are available to employers attempting to masculinize beauty for men. They hire women who already possess and display a heterofeminine habitus. It is true that female clients also tend to have their hair cut and styled by women, but these exchanges look and accomplish something different in men's salons. Adonis and The Executive build a brand around the sexualization of straight women, positioning them as tertiary objects of consumption and masculinizing "identity resources."[12] The women help to create and amplify a particularly classed gender experience for clients by fetching the men beer, ruffling their fingers through the men's hair, and ensuring the men their hair (or lack thereof) is attractive. Women interact with clients to reproduce class and racial distinctions on the shop floor,[13] and their labor ends up supporting men's socially sanctioned entitlement to women's sexual identities, bodies, and emotions.

Bringing together the sociology of consumption and the sociology of work, this book demonstrates how the organization of gendered labor supports a new consumer market. And by looking at women's roles in rebranding beauty for men, I argue that we can better understand how power informs the corporate production of men's beauty and the experience of creating more beautiful male bodies. Emotional labor, aesthetic labor, and physical labor together create a heteromasculine, middle-class brand image and consumer experience. I elaborate and retheorize these concepts by emphasizing the role of heterosexuality in aesthetic labor and touch-ing rules in physical and emotional labor. These rules help stylists to create loyal clients, and at the same time, these women make sense of their bodies, work, and identities in ways that protect them from feelings of degradation, exploitation, objectification, and commodification. When men appear as stylists and barbers, we see how this gendered labor operates differently to maintain the heteromasculinity of both clients and workers.

WHERE TO GO FROM HERE

Like with all research, this project tells only part of a larger story. Body prac-tices tend to look different by race, class, and sexuality,[14] and so the meaning of beauty consumption for men and the experiences of beauty workers who groom them are likely to vary across groups. How might salons differently deliver services in West Hollywood, a neighborhood with a prominent gay population and just a few miles from my field sites? What sort of classed, gendered, and racial philosophies underpin services at über high-end salons in Beverly Hills? Black barbershops highlight community in ways Adonis and The Executive do not,[15] and so scholars might ask: How do racialized and classed feeling and touching rules shape these communal relationships? How might customers and barbers make sense of their physical exchanges in black barbershops? What sort of bodily connotations and racial-ized gender relationships emerge in Latino barbershops? In white, blue-collar barbershops?

As more research on men's bodies emerge, it is important to consider how their diverse social locations translate into distinct corporeal con-sumer practices, and how race, class, gender, and sexuality come together differently to inform the labor practices that symbolically and contextually make men. The meanings and experiences of beauty service work and con-sumption are complicated and various, and while we know a lot about black women's rejection of white norms via the nurturing of natural hair,[16] and about white beauticians' negotiation of status while grooming professional women,[17] we know less about men in similar situations. There is room to study the bodily repertoires of men of color and the labor that makes these repertoires possible, as well as the emerging high-end hipster barbershops that acquaint young men with the nostalgia of homosocial spaces.

By studying men's salons, I hoped to capture the lived experiences of an understudied consumer and worker population, as well as the different ways gender informs the production of identities, status, and social hierarchies through everyday practices. I see studying men's aesthetic-enhancing practices (especially those other than typically hegemonic masculine practices like bodybuilding) as an avenue for exploring the reimagination, reorganization, and reproduction of gender as it plays out through interpersonal interactions, cultural symbols, organizational rhetoric, and structural ideologies. I encourage us to consider what happens when we replace women beauty workers with men. These men work in a female-dominated and feminized occupation where their heterosexuality might come under suspicion, and in which they navigate the work of emotionally and physically caring for others—work that usually supports biologized beliefs about women's natural propensities. I rely on Joshua, Ryan, and Randy to investigate the ways heterosexual aesthetic labor, feeling rules, and touching rules shape men and women's labor and relationships with clients, and what differences in how this work is organizationally required and interpersonally accomplished might teach us about power in the growing grooming industry. More of these men should be studied, and it is my hope that these concepts can help us to better understand processes of inequalities in other sorts of workplaces. How might touching rules play out in white-collar corporate settings, where women tend to occupy subordinate positions to men? How might men working as nurses or strippers utilize heterosexual aesthetic labor to form relationships with their patients or customers, and with their employers?

REFASHIONING BEAUTY WORK

Creating more supportive and less exploitive workplaces is not just a matter of firing one manager who discriminates when hiring employees or who institutionalizes sexist work requirements—although that would certainly help on a case-by-case basis. Social scientists instead understand that prejudiced practices and exploitive experiences are wide sweeping and are linked to larger structural inequalities. Inequalities are expressed in people's relationships with one another but informed by normalized cultural biases and larger hierarchies of power. The organization of labor at Adonis and The

Executive, for instance, is informed by deeply ingrained and often taken-for-granted social expectations that women are naturally nurturing and that men cannot control their libidos. The reproduction of social inequalities along the lines of gender, sexuality, class, and race are not guaranteed, though. Inequalities do not remain stable—or, at least, do not look the same—across time and place, and moments of resistance within different contexts provide insight into how social change might take place. Sociology shows that structures exist precisely because patterns in institutional and interpersonal behavior are observable, but people also have the ability to participate in resistant agency, whereby they express opposition to the status quo.[18] We might ask: What are the possibilities for transformation in men's salons? Can women empower themselves while also fulfilling organizational labor requirements? What might a contemporary labor movement among beauty workers look like?

Moments of resistance, pleasure, and alternative identity production reveal the ways women who groom men empower themselves within everyday interactions. They sometimes refuse to adopt the organizational ideologies of the salons and reject clients' claims to their emotional labor and heterosexual identities. When women call clients to tell them it is inappropriate to ask them out on dates, they draw boundaries around what they will and will not accept as legitimate worker-client interactions. When they create valued associations of women's beauty culture and women's homosocial relationships, they undermine an otherwise misogynistic grooming industry. Women can and do resist gender inequality on the job—the same inequality that places them in this type of work in the first place.

It is also significant that they express pleasure in many aspects of their work and fashion worthwhile identities. The psychological benefits of designing their own meaningful worlds are important to the workers' overall well-being. As Miliann Kang suggests, the social behavior of grooming allows workers to, at times, forge authentic selves within otherwise commercial exchanges.[19] By giving value to pleasurable labor experiences and human connections, and by forging dignified identities, people make their work significant and demand more equitable interactions with consumers. These small moments of resistance have the potential to snowball into change on a localized but organizational level. High-service men's salons like Adonis and The Executive rely on women workers to recruit a loyal clientele. Salons want clients to become attached to their stylists and nail technicians, and so these organizations are uniquely motivated to retain their employees. This dependence could destabilize typical organization-worker hierarchies to give workers more power in negotiating labor expectations.

Organizations have to get on board for bigger change. We need to see shifts in formal institutional labor requirements and informal workplace cultures, as well as a conscious dismantling of workers as commercial bodies. While it can be intimidating to imagine larger structural social change, it is perhaps easier to conceive of changes in individual corporate policies and marketing efforts that might alter worker-client relationships. While structures indeed shape our organizational cultures and everyday interactions between people, reform can take place on the ground.

Some labor scholars study service workers who are unionized, such as hotel employees,[20] or who are part of ethnic enclaves that rally to support their rights, such as Korean nail technician protests in Manhattan.[21] Yet there have been no recent social movements among hair salon workers in the United States. Hairdressers fought to be recognized as legitimate workers and businesswomen by the early twentieth-century National Recovery Administration, and they resisted government labeling of their work as unhygienic and unprofessional.[22] Women wrote to their state representatives to justify the private practice of doing hair, and customers supported better health conditions for women working with coloring chemicals in poorly ventilated spaces. Some male barbers even stood behind kitchen beauticians and other small-shop women entrepreneurs, who eked out a living for themselves and their families by pressing and styling their neighbors' hair. These movements followed the Great Depression, a time when the economic landscape was shifting, hairdressing was becoming a formal industry, and the Roosevelt administration was introducing exclusionary professional codes.

As we move out of the Great Recession, perhaps the time is again right for a larger beauty worker labor movement. They have seen what an economic downturn means for their industry, and despite a popular cultural sentiment of individualism, workers are creating collective identities around shared exploitation and fighting for labor rights. Although recent legislative measures have weakened unions in states like Wisconsin,[23] unionized fast food workers have organized walkouts to fight for a living wage.[24] The women at Adonis and The Executive complained of sore feet, aching hands and wrists, and exhaustion, and their personal relationships are compromised by long work hours. Some reported that management sends them home to change into more sexually alluring clothing, and informal gendered labor demands make women disproportionately responsible for doing exploitive labor. They identified these as personal rather than organizational and structural issues, but the current political environment around workers' rights, in tandem with organizational dependence on clients' loyalty to particular beauty workers, creates the potential for imagining a collective movement by and for women who groom men.

APPENDIX A

CLASS, GENDER, AND THE ECONOMY IN THE STUDY OF MEN'S SALONS

"The old-fashioned barbershop is undergoing a revolution, and as the format fades away, the men's hair salon is moving in to replace it."

—Chris Riddell, *Financial Post*, 2013

Men's salons are a growing phenomenon, with small luxury boutiques popping up across the country and the billion-dollar Regis Corporation getting in on the ground floor with Roosters Men's Grooming Center. As a mecca for corporeal aesthetic enhancement, Southern California is peppered with salons dedicated to the primping and preening of men. Many of these salons attract the attention of journalists looking for an interesting news peg to engage popular discussions of the meterosexual and assumptions about dissolving gender inequalities. With numerous salons from which to choose and the hope that managers would see me as simply another inquisitor interested in the hot topic of men's grooming, I had expected that securing field sites for my research would be relatively easy. The economic recession, however, made salon owners hesitant to grant me access to their shop floors, their employees, and, above all, their clients.

I found that the organizational protection of clients' class privilege at high-service men's salons created barriers to soliciting interviews and to otherwise talking with men about their consumer experiences. For some clients I was able to interview, their cultural capital actually made them sympathetic to my work and therefore willing interview participants. I discuss below how the economic recession shaped my study of men's salons, as well as how corporate preoccupation with reproducing clients' class status impacted my access to men on both organizational and interpersonal levels. Reflecting on how gender played out in this study, I also show how my research interactions with clients are evidence that the salons are successful in preserving men's heterosexual masculine identities.

AN "ELEVATED EXPERIENCE": PROTECTING SALONS, PRIVILEGING CLIENTS

The Economy

The Great Recession was in full swing when I embarked on research for this book.[1] It was 2009 and unemployment was on the rise with consumer spending slowing. A reported 9.3 percent of people in the United States were without jobs and an average of 10.9 percent of those living in and around Los Angeles did not have paid formal work.[2] Economic decline has devastating effects for already financially vulnerable people, but unemployment and the national housing bubble burst hit even white-collar workers previously considered "recession-proof."[3] The owners and managers of men's salons understood that the recession put them at risk of being trimmed from their clients' usual grooming repertoires, and these fears were not unwarranted. They were selling luxury services at a time when many people were tightening their purse strings, after all, and men could just as easily have their hair cut at a Supercuts or barbershop for a fraction of the price.[4]

Awareness of fiscal vulnerability made managers and owners of potential field sites hesitant to let me into their salons. After spending a frustrating two months trying to gain access to one salon, the owners decided they did not want me hanging around their clients. They were afraid my conspicuous presence as a woman in a men's salon would make their clients self-conscious, and that my approaching men for interviews would undercut their efforts to provide clients' a high-service experience of escape and relaxation. "Check back in a couple of months," the regional manager told me. "Perhaps [the economy] will be different then."

I eventually received permission to study Adonis and The Executive. Tyler, the owner of Adonis, seemed to revel in the media attention his salon had been receiving; he did not flinch when I asked to study and take photographs of the salon and to interview his employees. He appeared proud that I was interested in his salon and certain that it was the best place for me to investigate men's grooming. Veronica, owner of The Executive, was sympathetic to me as a graduate student. As a supporter of higher education and professionalization, she understood the pressures of scholastic requirements as well as the importance of doing research. She happily supported my study. Both Tyler and Veronica made it clear that while I was welcome to spend time in their salons and to talk with employees, their clients were off limits. Tyler did not want me interviewing clients because, as the salon's manager, Whitney, explained, Adonis focused on creating an "elevated experience" for men that did not include being studied.

Veronica was similarly hesitant to grant me access to her clients because she believed that men were cutting back on non-necessities like manicures and waxing. She explained that the recession was slowing business, as evident by the fact that men who "come in every two weeks now maybe come in every four, and whoever comes four is pushing it out to six to eight." Veronica brought up the impact of the recession on her business five times during the interview. "We've declined probably about 5 percent overall for the year due to clients getting laid off and not being able to afford to come here anymore," she said. Tyler and Veronica were careful not to take for granted their clientele at a time when men might be under financial pressure to downgrade to cheaper haircuts or to nix their manicures and facials altogether. They are highly invested in providing a first-class experience for men that distinguishes their salons from more economical options and entices clients to keep coming back. "You get what you pay for," stylists often explained, and Tyler and Veronica hoped men appreciated the pleasure, privilege, and privacy their dollar afforded them at the salons, despite the economy.

Class-Privileged Clients

The salons were structured to shield clients from stress and discomfort, and to provide them with an experience marked by privacy, personalization, comfort, and the naturalization of class entitlement. The owners saw being approached for interviews as potentially uncomfortable for clients, and they therefore explicitly limited this interaction. The well-to-do clients at Adonis and The Executive do not simply purchase haircuts and manicures; they also purchase physical and emotional interactions with women that reinforce their sense of affluence. Tyler and Veronica protected clients' personal space to justify their prices and services during the economic recession. This barrier to interviews meant that I had to get creative with data collection in order to gain access to men's salon experiences.

I used Yelp.com reviews to help flesh out my data on clients' opinions of, experiences in, and recommendations for men's salons.[5] These online reviews addressed many of the topics I was interested in, albeit much more briefly than afforded in an in-depth interview. Men reviewing their salons summarize what they like about their haircuts, detail their salons' amenities, comment on interactions with stylists, and explain what the salons can do to improve their experiences as men—or as class-privileged men, more specifically.

Luckily, after months of hanging around The Executive, Veronica allowed me to design and conduct a customer survey. A survey is quick, and so my asking men to fill it out while they waited for their appointments or exited the salon did not, in her opinion, infringe on the cultivated experiences she worked so hard to create for clients. I designed the survey to gather demographic information about what sort of men frequent The Executive: How old are they? What sort of jobs do they hold? How do they define their sexual orientation? I added open-ended questions to the survey, too, so that men could answer in their own words how they discovered The Executive and what it is they like and would change about the space and services. Some of the more interesting data revealed where men had previously gone for their haircuts, with some having moved around a bit but many coming directly from women's salons. Results from the survey are sprinkled throughout this book and help to give context to my interviews.

Soliciting survey participants put me in direct contact with The Executives' clients, some of whom showed interest in my research and volunteered verbal, on-the-spot explanations of how and why they became clients of the salon. In this way, collecting surveys from some men evolved into short informal interviews. Veronica granted me permission to, at the bottom of the survey, request the contact information of clients who were willing to participate in interviews with me at a later time. Over twenty men left their names and email addresses, and twelve of these men agreed to an interview, either face-to-face or by phone. Because these are busy professional men who live in a fast-paced metropolis, it was difficult to convince them to take the time to meet with me in person or to spend more than a half hour talking with me on the phone.

"Studying up" in the social order can pose distinct difficulties when collecting data. This is because people who occupy a privileged social status are used to controlling their interactions with others and having authority. In their study of global elites, sociologist Joseph A. Conti and philosopher Moira O'Neil found that respondents who hold status often feel entitled to question the legitimacy of the research and to interrupt or dismiss the researcher—sometimes avoiding participation altogether.[6] This was certainly the case in my previous research when a participant called my study "stupid" because he didn't see the point of interviewing men about their salons and their bodies.[7] Studying up can be riddled with difficulties since privileged people are not used to being objects of study or inquiry, are protective of their time, and are unlikely to make themselves easily available to the researcher. Conti and O'Neil found that limited time was a constant issue in setting up and conducting interviews with elites. Their participants were used to being paid for their time, and so the time they did give for interviews—no matter how short—felt to them like a "donation."

Socially advantaged individuals may also not feel as if participating in research will benefit them. Structurally disadvantaged participants are more likely to see the importance of research that explores racial, gender, sexual, or class inequalities, which limit their own opportunities for success and with which they struggle daily. They may understand research as something that is beneficial to them: they get to tell their story and hope that their lives will be bettered because of their participation—although betterment is not always the result.[8] It is not easy to access potentially stigmatized, vulnerable, or otherwise disadvantaged populations, but the blockades inhibiting the study of those with privilege are distinct and restricted my ability to conduct lengthy interviews with professional white men who made it clear they had little time (one man did a phone interview with me while he was overseeing the installation of audiovisual equipment; he shouted to me over the sound of construction so I could hear him and hung up prematurely). This sort of behavior limited my ability to create rapport with clients and ultimately the amount of data I was able to gather from them.

At the same time the clients' class privilege made it difficult for me to secure interviews with them, some men were willing to participate in an interview precisely because they had a privileged cultural capital. In his study of macroeconomists, social scientist Neil Stephens found that elites, specifically academics, had a particular willingness to participate in research.[9] The men in my study were not academics, but they were mostly college-educated and so understood requirements to conduct research projects and could identify with me as a "college student." Some of them were even University of Southern California alumni, while others were avid USC football fans or had children who were students at the university. My association with USC, an expensive private university, acted as a common denominator that connected me to some clients who were willing to do the interview.

RESEARCHER'S GENDER AND ORGANIZATIONAL GENDERING: AFFECTS ON RAPPORT AND DATA

As a woman, it was obvious that I was not a client of Adonis or The Executive. But I was also not completely out of place like salon owners had feared (see chapter 2 on the *specter of homosociality*). Men in fact did not often pay attention to me since the salons, although catering to a male clientele, were stocked with women workers. They sometimes even mistook me for a stylist or receptionist. When I passed out customer surveys at The Executive, I stood to the side of the reception desk and sipped iced tea while men leaving their appointments shifted their gaze between me and Brinn, trying to figure out who to pay. Since many beauty providers at The Executive spent their downtime congregating at the front of the salon—at Adonis they hung out in the break room—it did not look odd that I was standing around. Only when I approached men about filling out the survey did they seem surprised by my presence. One man waiting for his appointment asked me, "Are you applying for a job?" Negotiating this interaction was difficult since I had to explain who I was and why I was interested in studying men like him without making him self-conscious and thus compromising his potential participation in my study. At the same time, however, this conversation, and others like it, provided me with the opportunity to probe the client about his impressions of the salon.

It is true that clients might have spoken more openly with another man about certain aspects of their salon experiences, such as their pleasure in the objectification of heterosexually attractive female stylists.[10] Being a woman, though, allowed me to build rapport with the female beauty workers. Feminist epistemologists who advocate 'women study women' foresee just this: participants might relate to researchers via shared sex and/or gender. This does not mean there are not other things separating women, such as differences in race, class, and sexual orientation. But gender is particularly salient for women who groom men, in their narratives of work duties and work identities, and in their everyday interactions with me. They talked to me at length about their clients, relaying unflattering stories about balding men who wish to look like Brad Pitt and laughing about men who flirt with them. They gossiped about their clients as if I were a friend or colleague, and they seemed to assume that as a woman I could relate to their descriptions of men. "You know men!" they would say. They also understood why I would be interested in studying men's salons. The women often nodded while I described my research goals. They saw themselves as working on the cutting edge of the beauty industry and, like me, believe their work experiences shed light on interesting aspects of masculinity. Some women told me that curious friends and family quiz them about what it is like to work on men, and they recounted for me with practiced rhetoric many of the hetero-gendered aspects of their jobs.

At the same time gender helped me connect with the women beauty workers, I was always only a quasi-insider. I blended in during my ethnographic observations, but I was concurrently an outsider and rarely privy to private conversations between stylists who gossiped about clients in Adonis's break room, which was closed to me. I was not a hairstylist and did not have the 1,600 hours of cosmetology training needed to help around the salons with things like shampooing. During my 2007 research at the women's salon, Shear Style, I found that sweeping hair was assigned to apprentices, who had to have attended vocational school. My offer to do these things came across as an insult, an arrogant proclamation that I could do their jobs without training. Veronica was not interested in my volunteering to sweep up hair and stock supplies, because those jobs were reserved for the shoe shiner, Antonio, or for stylists in training.

Gender operated a bit differently in my interviews with men—both the clients and the male stylist and barbers. Randy, the only male barber at

The Executive, seemed a bit unprepared for my interview request, despite the fact that I had spent months observing the salon and interviewing other stylists. I think he was hoping I would disappear before I asked him to sit down and talk with me about what it was like to groom other men. He obliged me, though, and spoke with me at length during a break between clients. While he initially seemed unsure of how to answer my questions, he started to warm up to me halfway through the interview—"perhaps a little too warm," I recorded in my fieldnotes:

> Randy flirted with me. Much like my interviews with the men at Shear Style three years ago, Randy continually interrupted the interview to ask me personal questions. On the one hand, I believe participants should be able to ask questions of researchers, especially since we are asking them to answer similarly private and sometimes intrusive questions about their lives. On the other hand, it was clear to me that Randy's questions were flirtatious; he made a comment about just how lucky USC is to have such a "smart and good-looking woman" for a student. Unsure how to reply to this remark, I thanked him and continued with my interview questions.
>
> I offered to buy Randy a Starbucks coffee as a "thank-you" for participating in the interview. I had done this with other beauty workers I interviewed. When I went to pay the cashier, he reached in front of me and shoved a five-dollar bill into the cashier's hand. "You're not supposed to buy the drink," he said, suggesting that women do not treat men to coffee. For weeks after the interview, I caught Randy staring at me and lingering around when I was interviewing other people. The last time I saw him, he said: "Maybe we can hang out sometime." Was he asking me on a date?

While men's flirting with me was not as much of an issue during this project as it was in my past research,[11] it does represent an obstacle for many women who study men.[12] Conventional gender arrangements that elevate men as experts are undermined when women researchers ask them to be objects of scientific analysis. After all, "To open one's self to interrogation is to relinquish control and thus to put the masculine self at risk."[13] In their study of drag queens, gender scholars Verta Taylor and Leila Rupp found their status as highly educated and economically privileged women disrupted their participants' sense of male power, and to reverse this, the drag queens sexually subjugated them by yanking down Verta and Leila's tops to reveal their breasts.[14] There would be no doubt who the women were. While I can't be sure Randy felt threatened by being taken as an object of research, his comments emphasized our relationship as a gendered and heterosexualized one rather than as one of researcher and participant.

Making my interactions with Randy more complicated, I had to carefully negotiate the come-on of a participant that I could not afford to alienate. My ability to resist his heterosexualized definition of the situation was limited. Some scholars argue that face-to-face research is ideal for consciousness raising and resisting otherwise problematic discourses that draw from and sustain unequal relationships[15]—like those relationships that make men feel entitled to women's romantic attention. I decided to allow Randy's heterosexualizing behavior and remarks to go on uninterrupted. While this made me uncomfortable, I believe Randy's behavior resulted partly from feeling self-conscious during the research and thus gave me some insight into the gendered nature of both his work and the interview. It also meant, though, that I was capitalizing on his potential sexual interest in me and consenting to being a desirable woman rather than an authoritative researcher. This tension reveals the complex nature of research, whereby power is not solely the researchers' but wrapped up with and reflected in the relative social locations of the researcher and the participant. How power differences play out during in-depth interviews and ethnographic observations has important implications for the data as well as for the exploitation of participants, both of which feminist epistemologists are concerned with.[16] As a straight man that worked alongside women in a hair salon, Randy might have had something to prove in his interactions with me and so used the interview as an opportunity to demonstrate his heterosexuality.

I did not notice many differences between my interactions with the white beauty workers and those of color, but there was a particular awkwardness during my interview with Antonio, the Mexican immigrant shoe shiner who I mention in chapters 3 and 4. Antonio already occupied a marginalized location in the salon as an ethnic other whose job included kneeling at clients' feet and cleaning up after the beauty workers. He described his job as "disgusting" at times, and I rarely saw him interact with other employees. This social isolation gave him agency in deciding which jobs he did first—unless a client was waiting for a shoeshine—but it also situated him at the bottom of the salon's occupational totem pole. When I asked Antonio for an interview, he was reluctant to participate. I have since wondered if the ethnic and class differences between us compelled Antonio to eventually agree to the interview. His subordinated position at the salon meant he did not have a lot of power to refuse demands made on his time and labor from Veronica, clients, stylists, and, perhaps by association, me. I made sure Antonio was aware he did not have to answer any question that made him uncomfortable, and I hope the interview gave him an opportunity to claim his voice and otherwise empowered him to define his work and workplace identity in his own words.

Gender did not obviously cause problems in my interviews with clients. They did not flirt with me, for instance. I did suspect, however, that some of them were willing to "help" me out with an interview because I was a young woman. The ease with which I was able to interact with these men might also have resulted from the short and depersonalized character of the phone interview. In my past research, I found that men drew from "masculine resources"[17]—projecting heterosexuality, emphasizing age, and deploying humor—to protect their masculinity during potentially feminizing research.[18] The men's salon clients represented in this book did not utilize these tools to protect their masculinity. These are *men's* salons, after all, and the masculinization of these spaces are meant to make them feel as if they are doing something right as men by being there.

APPENDIX B
PARTICIPANT
DEMOGRAPHIC INFORMATION

TABLE B.1   Participant Demographic Information, Employees/Owner

Pseudonym	Sex	Age	Race/ Ethnicity	Position	Salon	Time at Salon/ Time in Industry
Connie	Female	24	White	Stylist	Adonis	9 months/7 years
Mary	Female	24	White	Stylist	Adonis	6 months/3 years
Jesse	Female	28	White	Stylist	Adonis	3 years/10 years
Gabrielle	Female	31	White	Stylist	Adonis	2.5 years/9.5 years
Joshua	Male	31	Latino/ White	Barber	Adonis	2 years/15 years
Trish[1]	Female	29	White	Massage Therapist	Adonis	10 months/7.5 years
Ryan	Male	24	White	Stylist	Adonis	2 years/5 years
Jackie	Female	25	White	Esthetician	Adonis	6 months/4 years
Patricia	Female	28	Latina	Stylist	Adonis	2.5 years/ 3.5 years
Emily	Female	21	White	Stylist	Adonis	1.5 years/1.5 years
Eva	Female	24	Latina/ White	Stylist	Adonis	2.5 years/5 years
Holly	Female	22	White	Stylist/Nail Technician	Adonis	1.5 years/4 years
Corey	Male	35	White	Owner/Stylist	Corey's Place	15 years/15 years
Veronica	Female	39	White	Owner/Stylist	The Executive	5 years/11 years
Isabel	Female	31	Latina	Stylist	The Executive	3 years/9 years
Faith	Female	29	White	Stylist	The Executive	6.5 years/7 years
June	Female	29	Asian	Stylist	The Executive	3 years/7 years
Joanne	Female	41	White	Stylist	The Executive	10.5 years/18.5 years
Aggie	Female	28	White	Stylist	The Executive	2 years/4 years
Whitney	Female	24	White	Manager/ Receptionist	Adonis	3 years/3 years
Elsie	Female	23	White	Stylist	Adonis	2 years/4 years *(continued)*

TABLE B.1   Participant Demographic Information, Employees/Owner (*continued*)

Pseudonym	Sex	Age	Race/ Ethnicity	Position	Salon	Time at Salon/ Time in Industry
Rea	Female	23	White	Stylist	Adonis	3 years/6 years
Bridget	Female	41	White	Esthetician/Nail Technician	The Executive	2.5 years/7 years
Loretta	Female	45	White	Nail Technician	The Executive	8 months/Not Reported
Roxy	Female	38	White	Barber	The Executive	5 years/10 years
Kendra	Female	35	Asian	Stylist	The Executive	1.5 years/2.5 years
Brinn	Female	24	White	Receptionist	The Executive	1 year/1 year
Martha	Female	60	White	Barber	The Executive	2 years/2 years
Randy	Male	31	White	Barber	The Executive	4 years/14 years
Antonio	Male	35	Latino	Shoe Shiner	The Executive	9 years/9 years
Julie	Female	20	White	Receptionist	The Executive	9 months/9 months
Colleen	Female	19	White	Receptionist	The Executive	1 year/1 year
Nell	Female	26	White	Stylist	The Executive	2 months/2 months (in training)
Mirabel	Female	20	White	Stylist	The Executive	2 months/2 months (in training)
Ruth	Female	30	Asian	Stylist	The Executive	2 months/1 year (in training)
Vicky	Female	26	White	Stylist	The Executive	2 months/8 years (in training)

¹ Every employee besides Trish identified as heterosexual.

TABLE B.2   Partcipant Demographic Information, Clients

Pseudonym	Age	Race/ Ethnicity	Salon	Education	Occupation	Income	Sexuality[a]
Calvin	51	White	The Executive	BS	Computer Work	130k	Heterosexual
Finn	32	White	The Executive	BS	Business Owner	Not Reported	Heterosexual
Dan	61	White	The Executive	JD	Judge	250k	Heterosexual
Gill	54	White	The Executive	BS/BA	Sr. VP Dev. Software	450k	Heterosexual
Lenny	63	White	The Executive	MA	Fitness Trainer	70k	Heterosexual
Alfred	52	White	The Executive	BS	Unemployed	——	Not Reported
Adrian	40	Latino	The Executive	Some College	VP/GM	100k	Heterosexual
Matthew	29	White	The Executive	BS	Accountant	100k	Heterosexual
James	48	White	The Executive	High School	Construction	100k	Not Reported
Warren	34	White	The Executive	MBA	"Mr. Mom"[b]	——	Heterosexual
Derek	27	Latino/ White	The Executive	BS	Software Analyst	60k	Heterosexual
Jonathon	39	Latino	The Executive	Some College	Civil Engineer	200k+	Not Reported
Noah	34	White	Adonis	PhD	Assistant Professor	61.5k	Heterosexual
Amit	27	Middle Eastern	Other	BA	Graduate Student	20k	Not Reported

[a] In cases where no sexual orientation is reported, participants identified as "male," "married," or told me, "I didn't answer the sexual orientation question, but I'm married."
[b] Previously worked in marketing.

NOTES

PREFACE

1. Kathy Peiss, *Hope in a Jar: The Making of America's Beauty Culture* (New York: Henry Holt and Company, 1998).
2. E.g., Steve Johnson, "Labels Come, Go, But Trendy Men Are Here to Shave," *Chicago Tribune*, July 28, 2004, http://articles.chicagotribune.com/2004-07-28/features/0407280033_1_metrosexual-hair-cuttery-sports-illustrated-swimsuit-issue; Warren St. John, "Metrosexuals Come Out," *New York Times*, June 22, 2003, http://www.nytimes.com/2003/06/22/style/metrosexuals-come-out.html.
3. For an exception, see Laura Miller, *Beauty Up: Exploring Contemporary Japanese Body Aesthetics* (Berkeley: University of California Press, 2006), on the gender of Japanese corporeal aesthetics.
4. Susan Bordo, *The Male Body: A New Look at Men in Public and in Private* (New York: Farrar, Straus, and Giroux, 1999), 217.
5. Kristen Barber, "The Well-Coiffed Man: Class, Race, and Heterosexual Masculinity in the Hair Salon," *Gender and Society* 22.4 (2008): 455–476.

INTRODUCTION

1. Glenn O'Brien unexpectedly left *GQ* in May 2015 over a contract dispute and was hired the following November as top editor by *Maxim* magazine. Alex Williams, "Glenn O'Brien Reinvents Himself (Yet Again)," *New York Times*, November 11, 2015. http://www.nytimes.com/2015/11/12/fashion/glenn-obrien-reinvents-himself-yet-again.html?_r=0.
2. Glenn O'Brien, "Manicures for Men?," *GQ*, July 8, 2009, http://www.gq.com/style/style-guy/grooming/200907/manicures-for-men; "Armpit Hair: To Shave or Not to Shave?," *GQ*, October 14, 2000, http://www.gq.com/style/style-guy/grooming/200010/shave-armpits; "Pomade and the Slicked-Back Look," *GQ*, May 14, 2001, http://www.gq.com/style/style-guy/grooming/200105/slicked-back-pat-riley-ed-burns. Condé Nast, the company that produces *GQ* (*Gentleman's Quarterly*), reports the magazine had 860,019 verified subscribers in 2015 and that 72 percent of the 7,000,000 total audience were men. The online "circulation demographics" show readers have a median household income of $72,213 and that 33 percent have a household income of $100,000+.
3. See Martha McCaughey, *The Caveman Mystique: Pop-Darwinism and the Debates Over Sex, Violence, and Science* (London: Routledge, 2008).

4. Kathy Peiss, *Hope in a Jar: The Making of America's Beauty Culture* (New York: Henry Holt and Company, 1998).

5. Raewyn Connell, *Gender and Power* (Stanford, CA: Stanford University Press, 1987); Michael S. Kimmel, "Masculinity as Homophobia: Fear, Shame, and Silence in the Construction of Gender Identity," in *Theorizing Masculinities*, ed. Harry Brod and Michael Kaufman (Thousand Oaks, CA: Sage, 1994), 119–141.

6. $6.2753 according to Euromonitor International, *Men's Grooming Products—US* (London: Euromonitor International, May 2008).

7. IBISWorld, *Hair and Nail Salons in the US—Industry Market Research Report* (Los Angeles: IBISWorld, August 2010).

8. On housework: Suzanne M. Bianchi et al., "Housework: Who Did, Does or Will Do It, and How Much Does it Matter?" *Social Forces* 91.1 (2012): 55–63; Scott Coltrane, "Research Household Labor: Modeling and Measuring the Social Embeddedness of Routine Family Work," *Journal of Marriage and Family* 62.4 (2000): 1208–1233. On men as secondary earners: Kristin Smith, "Recessions Accelerate Trend of Wives as Breadwinners," *Carsey School of Public Policy at the Scholars' Repository*, 2012, http://scholars.unh.edu/carsey/181. On stay-at home fathers: Noelle Chesley, "Stay-at-Home Fathers and Breadwinning Mothers: Gender, Couple Dynamics, and Social Change," *Gender and Society* 25.5 (2011): 642–664.

9. Tristan Bridges and C. J. Pascoe, "Hybrid Masculinities: New Directions in the Sociology of Men and Masculinities," *Sociology Compass* 8.3 (2014): 246–258. Bridges and Pascoe theorize a "hybrid masculinity" that symbolically rejects hegemonic masculinities at the same time it sustains existing hierarchies.

10. Kristen Barber, "The Well-Coiffed Man: Class, Race, and Heterosexual Masculinity in the Hair Salon," *Gender and Society* 22.4 (2008): 455–476.

11. Connell, *Gender and Power*.

12. Glenn O'Brien, "Male Facials," *GQ*, May 14, 2006, http://www.gq.com/style/style-guy/grooming/200605/facials-men.

13. "The New Business Casual," *GQ*, September 2010, http://www.gq.com/style/wear-it-now/201009/new-business-casual-september-gq-style#slide=1.

14. "The Man Bag Mans Up," *GQ*, October 2010, http://www.gq.com/style/wear-it-now/201010/man-bags-purse-briefcase-satchel-messenger-bag#slide=1.

15. Louis Williams, "The Relationship between a Black Barbershop and the Community That Supports It," *Human Mosaic* 27.1–2 (1993): 29–33; Earl Wright II, "More Than Just a Haircut: Sociability within the Urban African American Barbershop," *Challenge: A Journal of Research on African American Men* 9 (1998): 1–13; Earl Wright II and Thomas C. Calhoun, "From the Common Thug to the Local Businessman: An Exploration into an Urban African American Barbershop," *Deviant Behavior: An Interdisciplinary Journal* 22.3 (2001): 267–288.

16. While the corner barbershop is disappearing, upscale, throwback barbershops are emerging in urban areas. The new upscale barbershop harks back to a time when wealthy men saw their barbers for a pampering haircut, shave, and manicure, and embraces hipster masculinities that emphasize presumed gender egalitarianism and elaborately designed and confidence-inspiring beards and mustaches. The IBISWorld report on hair salons

notes: "Posh men's barbershops are popping up all over the country, luring men to a haircut and shave in more of a man-cave environment than a sitting-room environment." IBISWorld, *Hair Salons in the US—IBISWorld Industry Report oD4410* (Los Angeles: IBISWorld, February 2015), 8.

17. Barber, "The Well-Coiffed Man"; Tristan Bridges, "Bacon, Beards, and Beer: Feminist Reflections on Hipster Masculinity," *The Society Pages,* July 31, 2014, http://thesocietypages.org/feminist/2014/07/31/bacon-beards-and-beer-feminist-reflections-on-hipster-masculinity; David Coad, *The Metrosexual: Gender, Sexuality, and Sports* (Albany: State University of New York Press, 2008).

18. E.g., Luis Alvarez, *The Power of the Zoot: Youth Culture and Resistance during World War II* (Berkeley: University of California Press, 2009).

19. "High-service" bodily labor emphasizes pampering, emotional sensitivity, and relaxation, and is pleasurable, luxurious, and generally marketed to and consumed by white middle-class women. Miliann Kang, "The Managed Hand: The Commercialization of Bodies and Emotions in Korean Immigrant-Owned Nail Salons," *Gender and Society* 17.6 (2003): 820–839; Miliann Kang, *The Managed Hand: Race, Gender, and the Body in Beauty Service Work* (Berkeley: University of California Press, 2010).

20. Margaret Carlisle Duncan, "The Politics of Women's Body Images and Practices: Foucault, the Panopticon, and *Shape* Magazine," *Journal of Sport and Social Issues* 18.1 (1994): 48–65; Michel Foucault, *Discipline and Punish: The Birth of the Prison* (New York: Pantheon Books, 1975); John Germov and Lauren Williams, "Dieting Women: Self-Surveillance and the Body Panopticon," in *Weighty Issues: Fatness and Thinness as Social Problems,* ed. Jeffry Sobal and Donna Maurer (Hawthorne, NY: Aldine, 1999), 117–132.

21. Naomi Wolf, *The Beauty Myth: How Images of Beauty Are Used against Women* (New York: Random House, 1991).

22. See Julie Bettie, *Women without Class: Girls, Race, Identity* (Berkeley: University of California Press, 2003); Jeanine C. Cogan, "Lesbians Walk the Tightrope of Beauty: Thin Is In but Femme Is Out," *Journal of Lesbian Studies* 3.4 (1999): 77–89; Maxine Leeds Craig, "Race, Beauty, and the Tangled Knot of Guilty Pleasure," *Feminist Theory* 7.2 (2006): 159–177; Debra Gimlin, "Pamela's Place: Power and Negotiation in the Hair Salon," *Gender and Society* 10.5 (1996): 505–526; Mary Nell Trautner, "Doing Gender, Doing Class: The Performance of Sexuality in Exotic Dance Clubs," *Gender and Society* 19.6 (2005): 771–788; Rose Weitz, *Rapunzel's Daughters: What Women's Hair Tells Us about Women's Lives* (New York: Farrar, Straus and Giroux, 2004).

23. Candace West and Sarah Fenstermaker, "Doing Difference," *Gender and Society* 9.1 (1995): 8–37.

24. Kang, *The Managed Hand.*

25. Kimberly Battle-Walters, *Sheila's Shop: Working Class African American Women Talk about Life, Love, Race, and Hair* (Lanham, MD: Rowman & Littlefield, 2004); Paula Black, *The Beauty Industry: Gender, Culture, Pleasure* (London: Routledge, 2004); Frida Kerner Furman, *Facing the Mirror: Older Women and Beauty Shop Culture* (London: Routledge, 1997); Lanita Jacobs-Huey, *From the Kitchen to the Parlor: Language and*

Becoming in African American Women's Hair Care (New York: Oxford University Press, 2006); Julia A. Willett, *Permanent Waves: The Making of the American Beauty Shop* (New York: New York University Press, 2000).

26. Kristen Dellinger and Christine L. Williams, "Make-Up at Work: Negotiating Appearance Rules in the Workplace," *Gender and Society* 11.2 (1997): 151–177; Samantha Holland, *Alternative Femininities: Body, Age, and Identity* (New York: Berg Publishers, 2004).

27. For more on the pleasure and healthfulness of "beauty therapy," see Paula Black, "'Ordinary People Come Through Here': Locating the Beauty Salon in Women's Lives," *Feminist Review* 71.1 (2002): 2–17.

28. Foucault, *Discipline and Punish*, 25.

29. Jennifer Baumgardner and Amy Richards, "Who's the Next Gloria? The Quest for the Third Wave Superleader," in *Catching a Wave: Reclaiming Feminism for the 21st Century*, ed. Rory Dicker and Alison Piepmeier (Boston: Northeastern University Press, 2003), 159–170. Baumgardner and Richards challenge the notion that feminism and femininity are inherently oppositional; they argue that scholars and activists should embrace "girliness" and power as cooperative.

30. Nick Crossley argues that Cartesian ontology misrepresents the mind and body as separate and points to Maurice Merleau-Ponty's work as bridging this gap and laying the theoretical foundation for a "carnal sociology of the body." Here, meaning rises out of bodily interactions with the world and perception is not the inner representation of the outer world, but the result of engaging with the world: "Perception occurs in-the-world rather than the mind." Nick Crossley, "Merleau-Ponty, the Elusive Body, and Carnal Sociology," *Body and Society* 1.1 (1995): 46. See also Carol Wolkowitz, *Bodies at Work* (Thousand Oaks, CA: Sage Publications, 2006). A Cartesian perspective focussed on mind-body dualism elevates psychology while ignoring the centrality of the body as both organizing and organized by economic life.

31. Simon Goldhill, *Love, Sex, and Tragedy: How the Ancient World Shapes Our Lives* (Chicago: University of Chicago Press, 2004); Erik Gunderson, *Staging Masculinity: The Rhetoric of Performance in the Roman World* (Ann Arbor: University of Michigan Press, 2000); Joanne Entwistle, *The Fashioned Body: Fashion, Dress, and Modern Social Theory* (Cambridge: Polity, 2000); Colin McDowell, *The Man of Fashion: Peacock Males and Perfect Gentlemen* (New York: Thames and Hudson, 1997).

32. Gregory M. Zimmerman and Steven Messner, "Neighborhood Context and the Gender Gap in Adolescent Violent Crime," *American Sociological Review* 75.6 (2010): 958–980; Tristan Bridges, "Gender Capital and Male Bodybuilders," *Body and Society* 15.1 (2009): 83–107; Alan M. Klein, *Little Big Men: Bodybuilding Subculture and Gender Construction* (Albany: State University of New York Press, 1993); Michael A. Messner, "When Bodies Are Weapons: Masculinity and Violence in Sport," *International Review for the Sociology of Sport* 25.3 (1990): 203–220; Michael A. Messner and Donald F. Sabo, *Sex, Violence, and Power in Sports: Rethinking Masculinity* (Freedom, CA: The Crossing Press, 1994).

33. Messner, "When Bodies Are Weapons"; Michael A. Messner, *Power at Play: Sports and the Problem of Masculinity* (Boston: Beacon Press, 1992).

34. Leila J. Rupp and Verta Taylor, *Drag Queens at the 801 Cabaret* (Chicago: University of Chicago Press, 2003).

35. Barber, "The Well-Coiffed Man."

36. Also see Kristen Barber, "Styled Masculinity: Men's Consumption of Salon Hair Care and the Construction of Difference," in *Exploring Masculinities: Identity, Inequality, Continuity, and Change*, ed. C. J. Pascoe and Tristan Bridges (Oxford: Oxford University Press, 2015), 69–79.

37. Erving Goffman, "On Face-Work: An Analysis of Ritual Elements of Social Interaction," *Psychiatry: Journal for the Study of Interpersonal Processes* 18.3 (1955): 213–231; George Herbert Mead, *George Herbert Mead: On Social Psychology—Selected Papers*, ed. Anselm Strauss (Chicago: University of Chicago Press, 1934 [rpt. 1964]); Eviatar Zerubavel, "Islands of Meaning," in *The Production of Reality: Essays and Readings on Social Interaction*, 5th ed., ed. Jodi A. O'Brien (Thousand Oaks, CA: Sage Publications, 1991 [rpt. 2010]), 11–27.

38. West and Fenstermaker, "Doing Difference"; Candace West and Don H. Zimmerman, "Doing Gender," *Gender and Society* 1.2 (1987): 125–151.

39. The global north/global south reflects socioeconomic and political distinctions between North America/Western Europe/Australia/parts of Asia and South America/ Eastern Europe/Africa/the Middle East/developing Asia.

40. George Ritzer, *Explorations in the Sociology of Consumption: Fast Food Restaurants, Cards, and Casinos*, vol. 2 (London: Sage, 2001).

41. For instance, important work has been done on the exploitation of Barbadian workers who assemble computers sold in the United States and on young Chinese women who face dangerous conditions to make plastic beaded Mardi Gras necklaces. The computer user and Mardi Gras partygoer are largely absent from these labor accounts. Carla Freeman, *High Tech and High Heels in the Global Economy: Women, Work, and Pink-Collar Identities in the Caribbean* (Durham, NC: Duke University Press, 2000); *Mardi Gras: Made in China*, directed by David Redmon (New York: Carnivalesque Films, 2008), DVD.

42. Rachel Sherman, *Class Acts: Service and Inequality in Luxury Hotels* (Berkeley: University of California Press, 2007).

43. E.g., Christine L. Williams and Catherine Connell, "'Looking Good and Sounding Right': Aesthetic Labor and Social Inequality in the Retail Industry," *Work and Occupations* 37.3 (2010): 349–377.

44. For an exception, see Kjerstin Gruys, "Does This Make Me Look Fat?: Aesthetic Labor and Fat Talk as Emotional Labor in a Women's Plus-Size Clothing Store," *Social Problems* 59.4 (2012): 481–500.

45. Arlie Hochschild, *The Managed Heart: Commercialization of Human Feeling* (Berkeley: University of California Press, 1983).

46. This includes hairdressers, hairstylists, and cosmetologists and 660 barbers. U.S. Department of Labor, Bureau of Labor Statistics, "Occupational Employment and Wages: Hairdressers, Hairstylists, and Cosmetologists" (Washington, DC: Bureau of Labor Statistics, 2014); U.S. Department of Labor, Bureau of Labor Statistics, "Occupational Employment and Wages: Barbers" (Washington, DC: Bureau of Labor Statistics, 2014).

47. Dana M. Britton, "The Epistemology of the Gendered Organization," *Gender and Society* 14.3 (2000): 419.

48. See Joan Acker, "Hierarchies, Jobs, Bodies: A Theory of Gendered Organizations," *Gender and Society* 4.2 (1990): 139–158; Joan Acker, "Inequality Regimes: Gender, Class, and Race in Organizations," *Gender and Society* 20.4 (2006): 441–464.

49. See Kris Paap, *Working Construction: Why White Working Class Men Put Themselves—and the Labor Movement—in Harm's Way* (Ithaca, NY: Cornell University Press, 2006). One interview participant was in construction.

50. Barber, "The Well-Coiffed Man"; Lynne Luciano, *Looking Good: Male Body Image in Modern America* (New York: Hill and Wang, 2001).

51. For more on negotiating insider/outsider status in field research, see Teresa Brannick and David Coghlan, "In Defense of Being 'Native': The Case for Insider Academic Research," *Organisational Research Methods* 10.1 (2007): 59–74; Patricia Hill Collins, "Transforming the Inner Circle: Dorothy Smith's Challenge to Sociological Theory," *Sociological Theory* 10.1 (1992): 73–80; Pamela Cotterill, "Interviewing Women: Issues of Friendship, Vulnerability, and Power," *Women's Studies International Forum* 15.5 (1992): 593–606; Robert K. Merton, "Insiders and Outsiders: A Chapter in the Sociology of Knowledge," *American Journal of Sociology* 78.1 (1972): 9–47; and Nancy A. Naples, "A Feminist Revisiting of the Insider/Outsider Debate: The 'Outsider Phenomenon' in Rural Iowa," *Qualitative Sociology* 19.1 (1996): 83–106.

52. Telephone interviews can miss important contextual and nonverbal data, and the absence of visual cues can inhibit rapport between interviewers and participants. See Roger Shuy, *Linguistic Battles in Trademark Disputes* (New York: Macmillan, 2002); Neil Stephens, "Collecting Data from Elites and Ultra Elites: Telephone and Face-to-Face Interviews with Macroeconomists," *Qualitative Research* 7.2 (2007): 203–216. The lack of face-to-face interaction, however, can also make participants feel more relaxed and comfortable opening up to the interviewer about personal information. Gina Novick, "Is There a Bias Against Telephone Interviews in Qualitative Research?," *Research in Nursing and Health* 31.4 (2008): 391–398.

53. See Ronald E. Hallett and Kristen Barber, "Ethnographic Research in a Cyber Era," *Journal of Contemporary Ethnography* 43.3 (2014): 306–330.

54. Yelp.com is arguably one of the most popular and recognizable online review sites, and a search for high-service men's salons in Southern California resulted in fifteen salons. By including Yelp.com customer reviews of many different Southern California men's salons, I am able to expose patterns in how men describe their experiences of beauty consumption in masculinized spaces while also maintaining the anonymity of Adonis and The Executive.

55. Hochschild, *The Managed Heart*; Black, *The Beauty Industry*; Gimlin, "Pamela's Place"; Kang, "The Managed Hand"; Kang, *The Managed Hand*.

56. Kang, "The Managed Hand"; Kang, *The Managed Hand*.

CHAPTER 1 MEN AND BEAUTY

1. Ellis Cashmore, "David Beckham: Rise of the Metrosexual," *CNN*, May 17, 2013, http://www.cnn.com/2013/05/17/opinion/beckham-metro-symbol/.

2. Mark Simpson, "Ryan Lochte Manscapes for Hours—With Liberace's Razors," *MarkSimpson.com*, May 3, 2013, http://www.marksimpson.com/blog/2013/05/03/ryan -lochte-manscapes-for-hours-with-liberaces-razors/.

3. Mark Tungate, *Branded Beauty: How Marketing Changed the Way We Look* (London: Kogan Page, 2011).

4. Lynne Luciano, *Looking Good: Male Body Image in Modern America* (New York: Hill and Wang, 2001), 14.

5. Kris Paap, *Working Construction: Why White Working Class Men Put Themselves—and the Labor Movement—in Harm's Way* (Ithaca, NY: Cornell University Press, 2006).

6. Kristen Barber, "The Well-Coiffed Man: Class, Race, and Heterosexual Masculinity in the Hair Salon," *Gender and Society* 22.4 (2008): 455–476; Kristen Barber, "Styled Masculinity: Men's Consumption of Salon Hair Care and the Construction of Difference," in *Exploring Masculinities: Identity, Inequality, Continuity and Change*, ed. C. J. Pascoe and Tristan Bridges (Oxford: Oxford University Press, 2015), 69–79.

7. Kathy Peiss, *Hope in a Jar: The Making of America's Beauty Culture* (New York: Henry Holt and Company, 1998).

8. Joanne Entwistle, *The Fashioned Body: Fashion, Dress and Modern Social Theory* (Cambridge: Polity, 2000). Also see Joseph Roach's discussion on the sociocultural significance of nakedness and subordination, specifically in realtion to how Africans in the United States were presented bare-bodied on slave blocks. This nakedness further dehumanized slaves who were symbolically faceless and nameless. Joseph Roach, *Cities of the Dead: Circum-Atlantic Performance* (New York: Columbia University Press, 1996).

9. Entwistle, *The Fashioned Body*.

10. Peiss, *Hope in a Jar*, 23.

11. Entwistle, *The Fashioned Body*.

12. John C. Flügel, *The Psychology of Clothes* (London: Hogarth Press, 1930).

13. The dandy paid considerable attention to primping and preening, and yet his behavior and embodiment was markedly masculine. He was not to be confused with the "fop," a seventeenth-century pejorative term for a man who was overly concerned with his appearance. See Entwistle, *The Fashioned Body*. Most often a comedic character in English literature, the fop was overly decorated and "voluminous" in presence with exaggerated bodily gestures, and was mocked or pitied by public commentators for forfeiting "too much of his masculinity for the lure of the latest style." Colin McDowell, *The Man of Fashion: Peacock Males and Perfect Gentlemen* (New York: Thames and Hudson, 1997), 40.

14. McDowell, *The Man of Fashion*.

15. Entwistle, *The Fashioned Body*, 127.

16. McDowell, *The Man of Fashion*, 116.

17. Luis Alvarez, *The Power of the Zoot: Youth Culture and Resistance during World War II* (Berkeley: University of California Press, 2009).

18. Ibid., 53.
19. Quoted in Peiss, *Hope in a Jar*, 166.
20. Also see George Chauncey on gay men's use of fashion to signal sexuality in pre–World War II New York City. George Chauncey, *Gay New York: Gender, Urban Culture, and the Making of the Gay Male World, 1890–1940* (New York: Basic Books, 1995).
21. Peiss, *Hope in a Jar*.
22. Kenon Breazeale, "In Spite of Women: *Esquire* Magazine and the Construction of the Male Consumer," in *The Gender and Consumer Culture Reader*, ed. Jennifer Scanlon (New York: New York University Press, 2000), 226–244.
23. Michael S. Kimmel, "Consuming Manhood: The Feminization of American Culture and the Recreation of the American Male Body, 1832–1920," *Michigan Quarterly Review* 33.1 (1994): 7–36.
24. Breazeale, "In Spite of Women," 230.
25. Ibid.
26. Peiss, *Hope in a Jar*.
27. Ibid., 254.
28. Ruth Brandon, *Ugly Beauty: Helena Rubinstein, L'Oréal, and the Blemished History of Looking Good* (New York: HarperCollins, 2011), 105.
29. Peiss, *Hope in a Jar*, 12, 4.
30. Ibid.; Julia A. Willett, *Permanent Waves: The Making of the American Beauty Shop* (New York: New York University Press, 2000).
31. Barbara Ehrenreich and Arlie Hochschild unpack the ways contemporary global poverty undergirds women's migration into both formal and informal jobs as nannies, maids, and sex workers. Barbara Ehrenreich and Arlie Russel Hochschild, eds., *Global Woman: Nannies, Maids, and Sex Workers in the New Economy* (New York: Henry Holt and Company, 2004). Also see Pierette Hondagneu-Sotelo, *Doméstica: Immigrant Workers Cleaning and Caring in the Shadows of Affluence* (Berkeley: University of California Press, 2001).
32. Peiss, *Hope in a Jar*.
33. Pierre Bourdieu, *Distinction: A Social Critique of the Judgment of Taste* (Cambridge, MA: Harvard University Press, 1984).
34. Rubinstein married twice. The popular press referred to her first husband as "Mr. Helena Rubinstein." He took care of their children while Rubinstein grew her business both in Europe and eventually abroad in the United States. Her second husband, Russian royal Artchil Gourielle, was twenty-three years her junior and inspired her midcentury men's line, called simply Gourielle. Brandon, *Ugly Beauty*.
35. Karen Rosenberg, "An Art Trove Built on Mascara and Cold Cream: Celebrating Helena Rubinstein at the Jewish Museum," *New York Times*, October 30, 2014, http://www.nytimes.com/2014/10/31/arts/design/celebrating-helena-rubinstein-at-the-jewish-museum.html?_r=1.
36. Peiss, *Hope in a Jar*.
37. Robert L. Boyd, "Transformation of the Black Business Elite," *Social Science Quarterly* 87.3 (2006): 602–617; Robert L. Boyd, "Depletion of the South's Human Capital: The Case of Eminent Black Entrepreneurs," *Southeastern Geographer* 49.3 (2009):

251–266. Brandon, *Ugly Beauty*, cites Helena Rubinstein as the first woman millionaire in the United States.

38. Peiss, *Hope in a Jar*. Also see Willett, *Permanent Waves*, for criticism of Walker for selling hair-straightening products and refusing to talk about the racial implications of these products during press interviews.

39. Willett, *Permanent Waves*.

40. Brandon, *Ugly Beauty*; Peiss, *Hope in a Jar*; Willett, *Permanent Waves*.

41. Willett, *Permanent Waves*.

42. Ibid.

43. Ibid.

44. Brandon, *Ugly Beauty*.

45. Willett, *Permanent Waves*.

46. E.g., Debra Gimlin, "Pamela's Place: Power and Negotiation in the Hair Salon," *Gender and Society* 10.5 (1996): 505–526; Miliann Kang, "The Managed Hand: The Commercialization of Bodies and Emotions in Korean Immigrant-Owned Nail Salons," *Gender and Society* 17.6 (2003): 820–839; Miliann Kang, *The Managed Hand: Race, Gender, and the Body in Beauty Service Work* (Berkeley: University of California Press, 2010); Lanita Jacobs-Huey, *From the Kitchen to the Parlor: Language and Becoming in African American Women's Hair Care* (New York: Oxford University Press, 2006).

47. Peiss, *Hope in a Jar*; Willett, *Permanent Waves*.

48. Willett, *Permanent Waves*.

49. Peiss, *Hope in a Jar*.

50. Brandon, *Ugly Beauty*.

51. Peiss, *Hope in a Jar*, 117.

52. Willett, *Permanent Waves*.

53. Ibid., 112.

54. Christine L. Williams, "The Glass Escalator: Hidden Advantages for Men in the 'Female' Professions," *Social Problems* 39.3 (1992): 253–267.

55. Luciano, *Looking Good*.

56. C. Wright Mills, *White-Collar: The American Middle Class* (New York: Oxford University Press, 1951).

57. Luciano, *Looking Good*, 41.

58. Ibid., 59.

59. Ibid.

60. Willett, *Permanent Waves*.

61. Luciano, *Looking Good*, 84.

62. Ibid., 86.

63. Barbershops were also sex segregated until the 1920s, when "the bob" became both a trend and a sign of women's rising independence during the suffragist women's movement. Women flocked to the barbershop for their short haircuts, forming long lines down the sidewalk. Some barbers rejected women as clients and hung signs outside their shops that read, "For Men Only." Other barbers, though, embraced the financial rewards women's movement into the barbershop provided them. Willet, *Permanent Waves*, 42.

64. Ibid., 161.

65. Paula Black's book on the beauty industry shows that workers use the term "grooming" to distinguish men's bodily treatments from women's and to describe a "general standard of body aesthetics which is not related to vanity or beauty." Paula Black, *The Beauty Industry: Gender, Culture, Pleasure* (London: Routledge, 2004), 132.

66. Willett, *Permanent Waves*, 161.

67. Luciano, *Looking Good*, 138.

68. Ibid.

69. Ibid.

70. Susan M. Alexander, "Stylish Hard Bodies: Masculinity in Men's Health Magazines," *Sociological Perspectives* 46.4 (2003): 535–554.

71. Susan Bordo, *The Male Body: A New Look at Men in Public and in Private* (New York: Farrar, Straus, and Giroux, 1999).

72. David Coad, *The Metrosexual: Gender, Sexuality, and Sports* (Albany: State University of New York Press, 2008).

73. Ibid., 24.

74. Jen Doll, "New 'Retrosexuals' Really Just Metrosexuals with a Wardrobe Change," *The Village Voice Blogs*, April 7, 2010, http://www.villagevoice.com/news/new -retrosexuals-really-just-metrosexuals-with-a-wardrobe-change-6711384; Aaron Traister, "'Retrosexuals': The Latest Lame Macho Catchphrase," *Salon.com*, April 7, 2010, http://www.salon.com/2010/04/07/retrosexuals_silliness/.

75. Paul Harris, "Metrosexual Man Bows to Red-Blooded Übersexuals," *TheGuardian .com*, October 23, 2005, http://www.theguardian.com/world/2005/oct/23/gender .books.

76. Traister, "'Retrosexuals.'"

77. Michael A. Messner and Jeffrey Montez de Oca, "The Male Consumer as Loser: Beer and Liquor Ads in Mega Sports Media Events," *Signs: Journal of Women in Culture and Society* 30.3 (2005): 1879–1909.

78. Euromonitor International, *Men's Grooming Products—US* (London: Euromonitor International, May 2010); Euromonitor International, *Men's Grooming in the US* (London: Euromonitor International, May 2015).

79. Numbers reported in constant 2015 dollars. IBISWorld, *Hair and Nail Salons in the US—IBISWorld Industry Report 81211* (Los Angeles: IBISWorld, February 2015).

80. Brandon, *Ugly Beauty*.

81. Kristen Dellinger and Christine L. Williams, "Make-Up at Work: Negotiating Appearance Rules in the Workplace," *Gender and Society* 11.2 (1997): 151–177. Barber, "The Well-Coiffed Man."

82. IBISWorld, *Hair and Nail Salons in the US—Industry Market Research Report* (Los Angeles: IBISWorld, August 2008).

83. From 1992 to 2012, the number of barbershops dropped 22.5 percent to 3,797 nationwide, and the Bureau of Labor Statistics reported a total of 116,000 barbers in 2015. A 2013 uptick in barbershops to 3,948 might reflect new hipster barbershops and/or men's salons reporting as barbershops. This is compared to 76,203 beauty salons and 707,000 hairdressers, hairstylists, and cosmetologists. In 2010 barbershops accounted for a mere

3.1 percent of the $45 billion Hair and Nail Industry, and this included barbershop sales of both products and services. United States Census Bureau, County Business Patterns, "Data Tables by Enterprise Receipt Size: U.S., All Industries" (Washington, DC: U.S. Census Bureau, 2015); U.S. Department of Labor, Bureau of Labor Statistics, "Household Data Annual Averages: Employed Persons by Detailed Occupation, Sex, Race, and Hispanic or Latino Ethnicity" (Washington, DC: Bureau of Labor Statistics, 2015) U.S. Department of Commerce, Economics and Statistics Administration, "Census of Service Industries: Sources of Receipts of Revenue" (Washington, DC: Bureau of the Census, 1992).

84. IBISWorld, *Hair and Nail Salons in the US* (2010).

85. Ninety-three percent of Supercuts' revenue comes from haircuts, while the remaining 7 percent is from product sales. Across the United States, the chain provides approximately 100,000 haircuts, with an average cost of $17, and 1,200 color applications each day. Hoovers, A Dun and Bradstreet Company, *Supercuts, Inc.* (Short Hills, NJ: Hoovers, A Dun and Bradstreet Company, 2009); Hoovers, A Dun and Bradstreet Company, *Supercuts, Inc. Profile* (Austin, TX: Hoovers, A Dun and Bradstreet Company, 2015).

86. Great Clips does not offer coloring services and "caters to men, who comprise 70 percent of all their clients and prioritize reduced waiting times." Hoovers, *Supercuts, Inc. Profile.*

87. Ronald S. Barlow, *The Vanishing American Barbershop: An Illustrated History of Tonsorial Art 1860–1969* (St. Paul, MN: William Marvy Company, 1996); Christian R. Jones, *Barbershop: History and Antiques* (Atglen, PA: Schiffer, 1999).

88. Barber, "The Well-Coiffed Man."

89. Research on the black barbershop covers the racialized gender socialization of young black boys, the performance of black masculinity, black cultural aesthetics, and the barbershop as a place for racial politics. Clyde W. Franklin II, "The Black Male Urban Barbershop as a Sex-Role Socialization Setting," *Sex Roles* 12.9–10 (1985): 965–979; Alexander, "Fading, Twisting, and Weaving"; Bryant K. Alexander, *Performing Black Masculinity: Race, Culture, and Queer Identity* (Lanham, MD: AltaMira Press, 2006); Roopali Mukherjee, "The Ghetto Fabulous Aesthetic in Contemporary Black Culture: Class and Consumption in the *Barbershop* Film," *Cultural Studies* 20.6 (2006): 599–629; Melissa Victoria Harris-Lacewell, *Barbershops, Bibles, and BET: Everyday Talk and Black Political Thought* (Princeton, NJ: Princeton University Press, 2010).

90. Euromonitor, *Men's Grooming* (2015).

91. IBISWorld, *Hair and Nail Salons in the US* (2010).

92. Ibid.

93. NAILS magazine estimates men now make up 3 percent of nail salon clients—not including men who purchase manicures and pedicures at hair salons or spas. NAILS Magazine, *2014–2015 Big Book: Everything You Need to Know About the Nail Industry* (Torrance, CA: Bobit Business Media, 2015).

94. Regis Corporations is the parent company of Sally Beauty Supply, Supercuts, Vidal Sassoon, and other popular and widespread chain stores.

95. Hoovers, *Supercuts, Inc.*

96. www.razeformendeals.com. Since first conducting this research, Raze stores have been closed and the website removed.

97. According to an analysis of www.roostersmgc.com/salonlocator/default.asp, September 6, 2015.

98. Michael Quintanilla, "H-E-B Aisle Is for Guys Only," *Houston Chronicle*, January 27, 2010, http://www.chron.com/life/article/H-E-B-aisle-is-for-guys-only-1708148.php.

99. Euromonitor International, *Men's Grooming Products—US* (London: Euromonitor International, May 2008).

100. Ibid.

101. Bianca London, "Metrosexual Men Cost Their Partners £230 Every Year in Beauty Products . . . and It's All David Beckham's Fault," *MailOnline*, July 1, 2013, http://www.dailymail.co.uk/femail/article-2352279/Metrosexual-men-cost-partners-230-year-beauty-products-bid-look-groomed-like-David-Beckham.html.

102. Of the approximately 707,000 hairdressers, hairstylists, and cosmetologists, 665,994 are women, and the remaining 41,006 are men. U.S. Department of Labor, Bureau of Labor Statistics, "Household Data Annual Averages: Employed Persons by Detailed Occupation, Sex, Race, and Hispanic or Latino Ethnicity."

CHAPTER 2 ROCKS GLASSES AND COLOR CAMO

1. Adonis uses Redken Color Camo for Men, which is advertised by the manufacturer as a quick process chemical that covers gray to make men look younger.

2. Euromonitor International, *Men's Grooming in the US* (London: Euromonitor International, May 2015).

3. See Butler's work on the performativity of gender and West and Zimmerman on the role of social accountability in "doing" gender. Judith Butler, *Gender Trouble: Feminism and the Subversion of Identity* (New York: Routledge, Chapman & Hall, Inc., 1990); Candace West and Don H. Zimmerman, "Doing Gender," *Gender and Society* 1.2 (1987): 125–151.

4. C. J. Pascoe, *Dude, You're a Fag: Masculinity and Sexuality in High School* (Berkeley: University of California Press, 2007), 54.

5. For work on feminist theories of the cultural symbolic order, see Raewyn Connell, *Gender* (Cambridge, UK: Polity Press, 2002); Sharon Hays, "Structure and Agency and the Sticky Problem of Culture," *Sociological Theory* 12.1 (1994): 57–72; Pat Kirkham, *The Gendered Object* (Manchester, UK: Manchester University Press, 1996).

6. Harold Garfinkel, *Studies in Ethnomethodology* (Englewood Cliffs, NJ: Prentice-Hall, 1967); Suzanne J. Kessler and Wendy McKenna, *Gender: An Ethnomethodological Approach* (Chicago: University of Chicago Press, 1985); West and Zimmerman, *Doing Gender*.

7. Maxine Leeds Craig and Rita Liberti, "'Cause That's What Girls Do': The Making of a Feminized Gym," *Gender and Society* 21.5 (2007): 697. Dana M. Britton discusses the theoretical pitfalls of conflating sex composition with organizational gender. Dana M.

Britton, "The Epistemology of the Gendered Organization," *Gender and Society* 14.3 (2000): 418–434.

8. Michel Foucault, *Discipline and Punish: The Birth of the Prison* (New York: Pantheon Books, 1975).

9. Kris Paap, *Working Construction: Why White Working Class Men Put Themselves—and the Labor Movement—in Harm's Way* (Ithaca, NY: Cornell University Press, 2006).

10. Christin L. Munsch and Robb Willer, "The Role of Gender Identity Threat in Perceptions of Date Rape and Sexual Coercion," *Violence Against Women* 18.10 (2012): 1125–1146.

11. James W. Messerschmidt, *Nine Lives: Adolescent Masculinities, the Body, and Violence* (Boulder, CO: Westview Press, 2000); James W. Messerschmidt, "Becoming 'Real Men': Adolescent Masculinity Challenges and Sexual Violence," *Men and Masculinities* 2.3 (2000): 286–307.

12. Robb Willer et al. found that when men were told they are feminine, they "expressed support for war, homophobic attitudes, and interest in purchasing an SUV" and approved of "dominance hierarchies" (980). Robb Willer et al., "Overdoing Gender: A Test of the Masculine Overcompensation Thesis," *American Journal of Sociology* 118.4 (2013): 980–1022. Also see Catherine J. Taylor, "Physiological Stress Response to Loss of Social Influence and Threats to Masculinity," *Social Science and Medicine* 103 (2014): 51–59.

13. Kristen Barber, "The Well-Coiffed Man: Class, Race, and Heterosexual Masculinity in the Hair Salon," *Gender and Society* 22.4 (2008): 455–476; Lynne Luciano, *Looking Good: Male Body Image in Modern America* (New York: Hill and Wang, 2001); Paap, *Working Construction*.

14. Sharon R. Bird, "Welcome to the Men's Club: Homosociability and the Maintenance of Hegemonic Masculinity," *Gender and Society* 10.2 (1996): 120–132.

15. Anne Allison, *Nightwork: Sexuality, Pleasure, and Corporate Masculinity in a Tokyo Hostess Club* (Chicago: University of Chicago Press, 1994), 169.

16. Elizabeth Bernstein, *Temporarily Yours: Intimacy, Authenticity, and the Commerce of Sex* (Chicago: University of Chicago Press, 2007).

17. Frida Kerner Furman, *Facing the Mirror: Older Women and Beauty Shop Culture* (London: Routledge, 1997).

18. Julia A. Willett, *Permanent Waves: The Making of the American Beauty Shop* (New York: New York University Press, 2000), 1.

19. Earl Wright II and Thomas C. Calhoun, "From the Common Thug to the Local Businessman: An Exploration into an Urban African American Barbershop," *Deviant Behavior: An Interdisciplinary Journal* 22.3 (2001): 276. Also see W.E.B. Du Bois, "The Twelfth Census and the Negro Problems," *The Southern Workman* 29.5 (1900): 305–309; Clyde W. Franklin II, "The Black Male Urban Barbershop as a Sex-Role Socialization Setting," *Sex Roles* 12.9–10 (1985): 965–979; William Ransom Hogan and Edwin Adams Davis, *William Johnson's Natchez: The Ante-Bellum Diary of a Free Negro* (Baton Rouge: Louisiana State University Press, 1951); Sadye H. Wier and John F. Marszalek, *A Black Businessman in White Mississippi, 1886–1974* (Jackson: University of Mississippi Press, 1977); Louis Williams, "The Relationship between a Black Barbershop and the Community That Supports It," *Human Mosaic* 27.1–2 (1993): 29–33; Earl Wright II, "More Than Just a Haircut: Sociability within the Urban African American Barbershop," *Challenge: A Journal of Research on African American Men* 9 (1998): 1–13.

20. Ray Oldenburg, *The Great Good Place: Cafés, Coffee Shops, Community Centers, Beauty Parlors, General Stores, Bars, Hangouts, and How They Get You Through the Day* (New York: Paragon House, 1989); Ray Oldenburg, *Celebrating the Third Place: Inspiring Stories About the 'Great Good Places' at the Heart of Our Communities* (New York: Marlow & Co., 2001).

21. In his article on hipster barbershops, JC Reindl of the *Detroit Free Press* states that "The high-end vintage barbershop trend is raising prices and quality standards for guys seeking a trim and an old-school shave." JC Reindl, "Hipster Barbershops: Young Men Seek Some Old-Fashioned Grooming," *Detroit Free Press*, February 20, 2015, http://www.gosanangelo.com/lifestyle/hipster-barbershops-young-men-seek-some -oldfashioned-grooming_19965231.

22. Barber, *The Well-Coiffed Man*.

23. United States Census Bureau, County Business Patterns, "Data Tables by Enterprise Receipt Size: U.S., All Industries" (Washington, DC: U.S. Census Bureau, 2015).

24. Tristan Bridges, "A Very 'Gay' Straight? Hybrid Masculinities, Sexual Aesthetics, and the Changing Relationship between Masculinity and Homophobia," *Gender and Society* 28.1 (2014): 58–82.

25. Lawrence A. Wenner, "In Search of the Sports Bar: Masculinity, Alcohol, Sports, and the Mediation of Public Space," in *Sport and Postmodern Times*, ed. Genevieve Rail (Albany: State University of New York Press, 1998), 302. Also see Michael A. Messner and Jeffrey Montez de Oca, "The Male Consumer as Loser: Beer and Liquor Ads in Mega Sports Media Events," *Signs: Journal of Women in Culture and Society* 30.3 (2005): 1879–1909.

26. Joan Acker, "Inequality Regimes: Gender, Class, and Race in Organizations," *Gender and Society* 20.4 (2006): 443.

27. Michael A. Messner, "Sports and Male Domination: The Female Athlete as Contested Ideological Terrain," *Sociology of Sport Journal* 5.3 (1988): 197–211; Michael A. Messner, *Power at Play: Sports and the Problem of Masculinity* (Boston: Beacon Press, 1992).

28. Michael A. Messner, Margaret Carlisle Duncan, and Kerry Jensen, "Separating the Men from the Girls: The Gendered Language of Television Sports," *Gender and Society* 7.1 (1993): 121–137.

29. Peter F. Murphy, *Studs, Tools, and the Family Jewels* (Madison: University of Wisconsin Press, 2001).

30. Fallon Schlossman and Louisa Alter say of men's hair trends: "fewer men are concerned with being labeled 'metrosexual,' and are far more concerned with being labeled a slob." Fallon Schlossman and Louisa Alter, "Trend Alert: Men, It's Okay to Care About Your Hair," *WNYC*, July 23, 2015, http://www.wnyc.org/story/trend-alert-its-okay -care/.

31. Paula Black defines "grooming" as the practice of "maintaining a general standard of body aesthetic which is not related to vanity of beauty but to a regular maintenance

routine" (8). Paula Black, "'Ordinary People Come Through Here': Locating the Beauty Salon in Women's Lives," *Feminist Review* 71.1(2002): 2–17.

32. Arlie Hochschild, *The Managed Heart: Commercialization of Human Feeling* (Berkeley: University of California Press, 1983).

33. Cate Poynton, *Language and Gender: Making the Difference* (Geelong, Australia: Deakin University Press, 1985).

34. Murphy, *Studs, Tools*, 3.

35. Adonis offers service bundles to men at reduced prices. These bundles are "Party Crasher," "Black Tie Optional," and "Tuxedo Time" and contain various combinations of the following: haircut, facial, manicure, pedicure, and straight razor shave. Adonis also provides facials, including the "Signature" and "Deep Cleanse."

36. Murphy, *Studs, Tools*, 17.

37. Ibid.

38. I revised the Executive's motto to ensure anonymity while maintaining the sentiment of the original wording.

39. Poynton, *Language and Gender*.

40. The idea that men are naturally inclined toward math and spatial analysis is echoed in the 2005 speech by Harvard's then president, Lawrence H. Summers, who suggested women's underrepresentation in math and the sciences can be explained by their innate inabilities in these areas. Such biological explanations ignore social science research that shows gender bias, stereotypes, and discrimination in both education and the workforce are responsible for tracking girls and women out of science, technology, engineering, and mathematics. See Jacob Clark Blickenstaff, "Women and Science Careers: Leaky Pipeline or Gender Filter?" *Gender and Education* 17.4 (2005): 369–386; Yu Xie and Kimberlee A. Shauman, *Women in Science: Career Processes and Outcomes* (Cambridge, MA: Harvard University Press, 2003).

41. Pierre Bourdieu, *Distinction: A Social Critique of the Judgment of Taste* (Cambridge, MA: Harvard University Press, 1984).

42. See Tristan Bridges, "Gender Capital and Male Bodybuilders," *Body and Society* 15.1 (2009): 83–107.

43. Lee Kynaston, "Five Women's Beauty Products That Men Should 'Borrow,'" *The Telegraph*, October 11, 2013, http://www.telegraph.co.uk/men/fashion-and-style/10365171/Five-womens-beauty-products-that-men-should-borrow.html; "Pretty Handsome! More Men Buying Women's Beauty Products," *New York Daily News*, June 29, 2012, http://www.nydailynews.com/life-style/fashion/report-men-increasingly-buying-women-beauty-products-article-1.1104625; Bianca London, "Metrosexual Men Cost Their Partners £230 Every Year in Beauty Products . . . and It's All David Beckham's Fault," *MailOnline*, July 1, 2013, http://www.dailymail.co.uk/femail/article-2352279/Metrosexual-men-cost-partners-230-year-beauty-products-bid-look-groomed-like-David-Beckham.html.

44. Debra Gimlin, "Pamela's Place: Power and Negotiation in the Hair Salon," *Gender and Society* 10.5 (1996): 505–526.

CHAPTER 3 HETEROSEXUAL AESTHETIC LABOR

1. Anne Witz, Chris Warhurst, and Dennis Nickson, "The Labour of Aesthetics and the Aesthetics of Organization," *Organization* 10.1 (2003): 33–54.
2. Lynne Pettinger, "Gendered Work Meets Gendered Goods: Selling and Service in Clothing Retail," *Gender, Work, and Organization* 12.5 (2005): 460–478.
3. Molly George, "Interactions in Expert Service Work: Demonstrating Professionalism in Personal Training," *Journal of Contemporary Ethnography* 37.1 (2008): 108–131.
4. Mary Nell Trautner, "Doing Gender, Doing Class: The Performance of Sexuality in Exotic Dance Clubs," *Gender and Society* 19.6 (2005): 771–788.
5. Christine L. Williams and Catherine Connell, "'Looking Good and Sounding Right': Aesthetic Labor and Social Inequality in the Retail Industry," *Work and Occupations* 37.3 (2010): 357.
6. Chris Warhurst and Dennis Nickson, "Employee Experience of Aesthetic Labour in Retail and Hospitality," *Work, Employment, and Society* 21.1 (2007): 103–120; Chris Warhurst and Dennis Nickson, "'Who's Got the Look?' Emotional, Aesthetic and Sexualized Labour in Interactive Services," *Gender, Work, and Organization* 16.3 (2009): 385–404.
7. For discussion of habitus, see Pierre Bourdieu, *Distinction: A Social Critique of the Judgment of Taste* (Cambridge, MA: Harvard University Press, 1984).
8. Williams and Connell, "'Looking Good and Sounding Right.'"
9. Christine L. Williams, *Inside Toyland: Working, Shopping, and Social Inequality* (Berkeley: University of California Press, 2006). As an example of this type of discrimination, Abercrombie & Fitch was famously accused of using discriminatory hiring practices in an effort to uphold a narrowly defined and exclusionary corporate "look." A class action lawsuit filed in 2003, *Gonzalez v. Abercrombie & Fitch*, charged the retailer with terminating and refusing to hire applicants and employees based on their race and ethnicity. The retailer settled for approximately $50 million in 2005 and was court ordered to institute diversity-promoting policies.
10. Lisa Adkins, "Mobile Desire: Aesthetics, Sexuality, and the 'Lesbian' at Work," *Sexualities* 3.2 (2000): 212. Also see Patti A. Giuffre, Kirsten Dellinger, and Christine L. Williams, "No Retribution for Being Gay?: Inequality in Gay-Friendly Workplaces," *Sociological Spectrum* 28.3 (2008): 254–277; Christine L. Williams, Patti A. Giuffre, and Kirsten Dellinger, "The Gay-Friendly Closet," *Sexuality Research and Social Policy: Journal of NSRC* 6.1 (2009): 29–45.
11. Adkins, "Mobile Desire."
12. C. J. Pascoe, *Dude, You're a Fag: Masculinity and Sexuality in High School* (Berkeley: University of California Press, 2007), 183.
13. Patricia Hill Collins, "Learning from the Outsider Within: The Sociological Significance of Black Feminist Thought," *Social Problems* 33.6 (1986): 14–19. Collins argues that black domestics who labor in the homes of whites are uniquely positioned as quasi-insiders who never truly belong. This "outsider-within" status makes them privy to the operations of white privilege in a way whites are not. Privilege is often invisible to those who hold it, and so men tend to not see how they are

advantaged by gender, whites by race, straights by sexuality, and so forth; Michael S. Kimmel and Abby L. Ferber, eds., *Privilege* (Boulder, CO: Westview Press, 2003). Peggy McIntosh refers to this as the invisible "knapsack of privilege." Peggy McIntosh, "White Privilege: Unpacking the Invisible Knapsack," *Peace and Freedom*, 1989, http://www.areteadventures.com/articles/white_privilege_unpacking_the_invisble_napsack.pdf.

14. For a discussion of women and rewards for makeup at work, see Kristen Dellinger and Christine L. Willliams, "Make-Up at Work: Negotiating Appearance Rules in the Workplace," *Gender and Society* 11.2 (1997): 151–177.

15. In their study of high-end retail, "'Looking Good and Sounding Right,'" Williams and Connell argue that hiring ready-made employees instead of participating in costly training practices is part of the historical transformation of labor that highlights efficiency and places the risk of hiring and firing in the hands of employees. Warhurst and Nickson contend that corporations demanding aesthetic labor may still find themselves developing employees' appearances to make sure workers fit the brand image at all times ("'Who's Got the Look?'").

16. Bryant K. Alexander, "Fading, Twisting, and Weaving: An Interpretive Ethnography of the Black Barbershop as Cultural Space," *Qualitative Inquiry* 9.1 (2003): 105–128. In his reflection on the black barbershop, Alexander discusses the pleasure of being touched by the barber and the homophobia that forces this pleasure underground.

17. Susan Bordo, *The Male Body: A New Look at Men in Public and in Private* (New York: Farrar, Straus, and Giroux, 1999).

18. Trautner, "Doing Gender, Doing Class." In her study of working- and upper-class strip clubs, Trautner shows that sexual and class aesthetics are inseparable.

19. Pascoe, *Dude, You're a Fag.*

20. Gayle S. Rubin, "Thinking Sex: Notes for a Radical Theory of the Politics of Sexuality," in *The Lesbian and Gay Studies Reader*, ed. Harry Abelove, Michele Aina Barale, and David M. Halperin (New York: Routledge, 1984), 13.

21. Raewyn Connell, *Masculinities* (Berkeley: University of California Press, 1995), 77.

22. See Sharon R. Bird, "Welcome to the Men's Club: Homosociability and the Maintenance of Hegemonic Masculinity," *Gender and Society* 10.2 (1996): 120–132; Michael S. Kimmel, "Masculinity as Homophobia: Fear, Shame, and Silence in the Construction of Gender Identity," in *Theorizing Masculinities*, ed. Harry Brod and Michael Kaufman (Thousand Oaks, CA: Sage, 1994), 119–141.

23. Trautner, "Doing Gender, Doing Class."

24. Kristen Barber, "The Well-Coiffed Man: Class, Race, and Heterosexual Masculinity in the Hair Salon," *Gender and Society* 22.4 (2008): 455–476; Kristen Barber, "Styled Masculinity: Men's Consumption of Salon Hair Care and the Construction of Difference," in *Exploring Masculinities: Identity, Inequality, Continuity, and Change*, ed. C. J. Pascoe and Tristan Bridges (Oxford: Oxford University Press, 2015), 69–79.

25. Ulla Forseth, "Gender Matters? Exploring How Gender Is Negotiated in Service Encounters," *Gender, Work, and Organization* 12.5 (2005): 447.

26. Forseth, "Gender Matters?"

27. Eileen M. Otis, "The Dignity of Working Women: Service, Sex, and the Labor Politics of Localization in China's City of Eternal Spring," *American Behavioral Scientist* 52.3 (2008): 360.

28. E.g., Debra Gimlin, "Pamela's Place: Power and Negotiation in the Hair Salon," *Gender and Society* 10.5 (1996): 505–526; Miliann Kang, "The Managed Hand: The Commercialization of Bodies and Emotions in Korean Immigrant-Owned Nail Salons," *Gender and Society* 17.6 (2003): 820–839; Miliann Kang, *The Managed Hand: Race, Gender, and the Body in Beauty Service Work* (Berkeley: University of California Press, 2010).

29. E.g., Otis, "The Dignity of Working Women"; Rachel Sherman, *Class Acts: Service and Inequality in Luxury Hotels* (Berkeley: University of California Press, 2007).

30. Sarah Oerton, "Bodywork Boundaries: Power, Politics, and Professionalism in Therapeutic Massage," *Gender, Work, and Organization* 11.5 (2004): 544–565; Sarah Oerton and Joanne Phoenix, "Sex/Body Work: Discourses and Practices," *Sexualities* 4.4 (2001): 387–412.

31. Also see Gimlin, "Pamela's Place."

32. Oerton, "Bodywork Boundaries," 555, 556.

33. For a discussion of symbolic boundary formation in hotel service work, see Sherman, *Class Acts.*

34. Rosabeth Moss Kanter, *Men and Women of the Corporation* (New York: Basic Books, 1977).

35. Barbara A. Gutek et al., "Sexuality and the Workplace," *Basic and Applied Social Psychology* 1.3 (1980): 255–265; Catherine A. MacKinnon, *Sexual Harassment of Working Women* (New Haven, CT: Yale University Press, 1979).

36. Kristen Dellinger and Christine L. Williams, "The Locker Room and the Dorm Room: Workplace Norms and Magazine Editing," *Social Problems* 49.2 (2002): 242–257; Christine L. Williams, Patti A. Giuffre, and Kristen Dellinger, "Sexuality in the Workplace: Organizational Control, Sexual Harassment, and the Pursuit of Pleasure," *Annual Review of Sociology* 25.1 (1999): 73–93.

37. Patti A. Giuffre and Christine L. Williams, "Boundary Lines: Labeling Sexual Harassment in Restaurants," *Gender and Society* 8.3 (1994): 378–401.

38. Rhacel Parreñas, "Hostess Work: Negotiating the Morals of Money and Sex," *Economic Sociology of Work*, vol. 18 of *Research in the Sociology of Work*, ed. Nina Bandelj (Bingley, UK: Emerald, 2009), 216.

39. Arlie Hochschild, *The Managed Heart: Commercialization of Human Feeling* (Berkeley: University of California Press, 1983).

40. Steve Taylor and Melissa Tyler, "Emotional Labour and Sexual Difference in the Airline Industry," *Work, Employment, and Society* 14.1 (2000): 77–95; Claire Williams, "Sky Service: The Demands of Emotional Labour in the Airline Industry," *Gender, Work, and Organization* 10.5 (2003): 513–550.

41. Kang, "The Managed Hand"; Kang, *The Managed Hand.*

42. In her study of Chinese luxury hotel workers, Eileen M. Otis finds that women respond to threats to their dignity by "embracing and elaborating professional protocols." *Markets and Bodies: Women, Service Work, and the Making of Inequality in China* (Stanford, CA: Stanford University Press, 2011), 33.

43. Amy M. Denissen, "Crossing the Line: How Women in the Building Trades Interpret and Respond to Sexual Conduct at Work," *Journal of Contemporary Ethnography* 39.3 (2010): 297–327.

44. "Mother I'd Like to Fuck."

45. Giuffre and Williams, "Boundary Lines."

46. Dellinger and Williams, "The Locker Room and the Dorm Room."

47. Martha McCaughey, *The Caveman Mystique: Pop-Darwinism and the Debates Over Sex, Violence, and Science* (London: Routledge, 2008). McCaughey unpacks popularized Darwinian ideas about men and sexuality. The image of the caveman, she says, is reimagined; instead of wearing fur or carrying a club, he is dressed in ties and vests. At the same time he embodies class privilege, he is also seen as biologically sexually impulsive and can't be blamed for his rampant attitudes about and aggressions toward women.

48. Teela Sanders, "Controllable Laughter: Managing Sex Work through Humour," *Sociology* 38.2 (2004): 273–291.

49. Barbara J. Risman, "Gender as a Social Structure: Theory Wrestling with Activism," *Gender and Society* 18.4 (2004): 429–450.

CHAPTER 4   HAIR CARE

1. This vignette exemplifies interactions between women working at The Executive and their clients and is comprised of details from my direct observations at this salon and stylists' interviews. Similar interactions occurred at Adonis.

2. Robin Leidner, *Fast Food, Fast Talk: Service Work and the Routinization of Everyday Life* (Berkeley: University of California Press, 1993). Leidner uses "interactive service work" to emphasize that the worker-customer interaction—or treatment of the customer—is itself a corporate product.

3. Heather Ferguson Bulan, Rebecca J. Erickson, and Amy S. Wharton, "Doing for Others on the Job: The Affective Requirements of Service Work, Gender, and Emotional Well-Being," *Social Problems* 44.2 (1997): 235–256.

4. For more on flight attendants, see Arlie Hochschild, *The Managed Heart: Commercialization of Human Feeling* (Berkeley: University of California Press, 1983); Steve Taylor and Melissa Tyler, "Emotional Labour and Sexual Difference in the Airline Industry," *Work, Employment, and Society* 14.1 (2000): 77–95; Claire Williams, "Sky Service: The Demands of Emotional Labour in the Airline Industry," *Gender, Work, and Organization* 10.5 (2003): 513–550.

5. Karla A. Erickson, "To Invest or Detach? Coping Strategies and Workplace Culture in Service Work," *Symbolic Interaction* 27.4 (2004): 549–572; Karla A. Erickson, *The Hungry Cowboy: Service and Community in a Neighborhood Restaurant* (Jackson: University Press of Mississippi, 2009); Karla A. Erickson and Jennifer L. Pierce, "Farewell to the Organization Man: The Feminization of Loyalty in High-End and Low-End Service Jobs," *Ethnography* 6.3 (2005): 283–313; Ray Oldenburg, *The Great Good Place: Cafés, Coffee Shops, Community Centers, Beauty Parlors, General Stores, Bars, Hangouts, and How They Get You Through the Day* (New York: Paragon House, 1989).

6. Teela Sanders, Rachel Lara Cohen, and Kate Hardy, "Hairdressing/Undressing: Comparing Labour Relations in Self-Employed Body Work," in *Body/Sex/Work: Intimate, Embodied, and Sexualised Labour*, ed. Carol Wolkowitz, Rachel Lara Cohen, Teela Sanders, and Kate Hardy (London: Palgrave Macmillan, 2013), 110–126.

7. Hochschild, *The Managed Heart*. Paula Black, *The Beauty Industry: Gender, Culture, Pleasure* (London: Routledge, 2004); Frida Kerner Furman, *Facing the Mirror: Older Women and Beauty Shop Culture* (London: Routledge, 1997); Ursula Sharma and Paula Black, "Look Good, Feel Better: Beauty Therapy as Emotional Labour," *Sociology* 35.4 (2001): 913–931. Debra Gimlin, "Pamela's Place: Power and Negotiation in the Hair Salon," *Gender and Society* 10.5 (1996): 505–526; Tracey Yeadon-Lee, "Doing Identity with Style: Service Interaction, Work Practices, and the Construction of 'Expert' Status in the Contemporary Hair Salon," *Sociological Research Online* 17.4 (2012). doi: 10.5153/sro.2726.

8. Miliann Kang, "The Managed Hand: The Commercialization of Bodies and Emotions in Korean Immigrant-Owned Nail Salons," *Gender and Society* 17.6 (2003): 820–839; Miliann Kang, *The Managed Hand: Race, Gender, and the Body in Beauty Service Work* (Berkeley: University of California Press, 2010).

9. Hochschild, *The Managed Heart*. Also see Adia Harvey Wingfield, "Are Some Emotions Marked 'Whites Only'? Racialized Feeling Rules in Professional Workplaces," *Social Problems* 57.2 (2010): 251–268; Kathryn J. Lively, "Reciprocal Emotion Management: Working Together to Maintain Stratification in Private Law Firms," *Work and Occupations* 27.1 (2000): 32–63.

10. Hairapy, a morpheme of hair and therapy, highlights the emotional labor tied to beauty work. "We definitely are hairapists," said Janine, a 2008 contestant on the reality show *Shear Genius*, where stylists are judged on their abilities to deliver precision and panache to the heads of hair models. "It's like, they get—I think that's why a lot of us charge so much for haircuts. It's a two-for-one. You're really saving time and money with getting your hair done and a therapy session out of the way."

11. Kang, "The Managed Hand"; Kang, *The Managed Hand*; Rachel Sherman, *Class Acts: Service and Inequality in Luxury Hotels* (Berkeley: University of California Press, 2007).

12. Jennifer L. Pierce, *Gender Trials: Emotional Lives in Contemporary Law Firms* (Berkeley: University of California Press, 1996).

13. Joan Acker, "Hierarchies, Jobs, Bodies: A Theory of Gendered Organizations," *Gender and Society* 4.2 (1990): 139–158; Joan Acker, "Inequality Regimes: Gender, Class, and Race in Organizations," *Gender and Society* 20.4 (2006): 441–464.

14. This idea reinforces rather than challenges gender dichotomies and the feminine characterization of the occupation. This dichotomy is made salient as especially white men who enter these jobs are tracked up to administration via a glass escalator, encouraged by others to seek further education, and offered promotions over female colleagues. They might find themselves institutionally or interpersonally discouraged from fulfilling the caring aspects of their jobs in order to appear masculine: men who nurse lift patients more often than bathe them, for example. Adia Harvey Wingfield, "Racializing the Glass Escalator: Reconsidering Men's Experiences with Women's Work," *Gender*

and Society 23.1 (2009): 5–26; Christine L. Williams, "The Glass Escalator: Hidden Advantages for Men in the 'Female' Professions," *Social Problems* 39.3 (1992): 253–267.

15. Harvey Wingfield, "Racializing the Glass Escalator"; Williams, "The Glass Escalator."

16. Hochschild, *The Managed Heart*, 56.

17. Acker, "Inequality Regimes."

18. For a look at nonheteronormative work cultures, see Kristen Schilt, *Just One of the Guys? Transgender Men and the Persistence of Gender Inequality* (Chicago: University of Chicago Press, 2010). For a discussion of heteronormative assumptions in the workplace, see Adia Harvey Wingfield, *No More Invisible Man: Race and Gender in Men's Work* (Philadelphia: Temple University Press, 2013).

19. Commissions range from 30–45 percent of the service price, depending on the salon and how long a beauty provider has been working there.

20. Pierce, *Gender Trials*, 58.

21. Sharon R. Bird, "Welcome to the Men's Club: Homosociability and the Maintenance of Hegemonic Masculinity," *Gender and Society* 10.2 (1996): 120–132; C. J. Pascoe, *Dude, You're a Fag: Masculinity and Sexuality in High School* (Berkeley: University of California Press, 2007).

22. Geoffrey Greif, *Buddy System: Understanding Male Friendships* (Oxford: Oxford University Press, 2008), 6.

23. Jeffrey A. Hall, "Sex Differences in Friendship Expectations: A Meta-Analysis," *Journal of Social and Personal Relationships* 28.6 (2011): 723–747.

24. Brant R. Burleson, "A Different Voice on Different Cultures: Illusion and Reality in the Study of Sex Differences in Personal Relationships," *Personal Relationships* 4.3 (2005): 229–241; Miller McPherson, Lynn Smith-Lovin, and Matthew E. Brashears, "Social Isolation in America: Changes in Core Discussion Networks over Two Decades," *American Sociological Review* 71.3 (2006): 353–375.

25. Lisa Wade, "American Men's Hidden Crisis: They Need More Friends!" *Salon,* December 7, 2013, http://www.salon.com/2013/12/08/american_mens_hidden_crisis _they_need_more_friends/.

26. Viviana A. Zelizer, *The Purchase of Intimacy* (Princeton, NJ: Princeton University Press, 2007), 5, 28.

27. Kristen Barber, "The Well-Coiffed Man: Class, Race, and Heterosexual Masculinity in the Hair Salon," *Gender and Society* 22.4 (2008): 467.

28. Martin O'Brien, "*The Managed Heart* Revisited: Health and Social Control," *Sociological Review* 42.3 (1994): 393–413.

29. Leidner, *Fast Food, Fast Talk.*

30. For a context specific exception, see Tristan Bridges, "A Very 'Gay' Straight? Hybrid Masculinities, Sexual Aesthetics, and the Changing Relationship between Masculinity and Homophobia," *Gender and Society* 28.1 (2014): 58–82.

31. Bird, "Welcome to the Men's Club"; Pierette Hondangeu-Sotelo and Michael A. Messner, "Gender Displays and Men's Power: The 'New Man' and the Mexican Immigrant Man," in *Theorizing Masculinities*, ed. Harry Brod and Michael Kaufman (Thousand Oaks, CA: Sage Publications, 1994), 200–218.

32. Barber, "The Well-Coiffed Man."

33. Demetrakis Z. Demetriou, "Connell's Concept of Hegemonic Masculinity: A Critique," *Theory and Society* 30.3 (2001): 337–361; Antonio Gramsci, *Selections from the Prison Notebooks*, ed. Quintin Hoare and Geoffrey Nowell Smith (New York: International Publishers, 1971); Tristan Bridges and C. J. Pascoe, "Hybrid Masculinities: New Directions in the Sociology of Men and Masculinities," *Sociology Compass* 8.3 (2014): 246–258.

34. Demetriou, "Connell's Concept," 349.

35. Bridges and Pascoe, "Hybrid Masculinities."

36. Arthur E. Thomas, "Future Shock from a Black Perspective," *Theory into Practice* 20.4 (1981): 237–244.

37. Timothy Bates, William E. Jackson III, and James H. Johnson Jr., "Introduction: Advancing Research on Minority Entrepreneurship," *Annals of the American Academy of Political and Social Science* 613 (2007): 12.

38. E.g., Dorothy E. Smith, "Women's Perspectives as a Radical Critique of Sociology," in *Feminism and Methodology: Social Science Issues*, ed. Sandra Harding (Bloomington: Indiana University Press, 2004), 84–96.

39. See Carol Wolkowitz, *Bodies at Work* (Thousand Oaks, CA: Sage Publications, 2006), 150.

40. Kris Paap, *Working Construction: Why White Working Class Men Put Themselves— and the Labor Movement—in Harm's Way* (Ithaca, NY: Cornell University Press, 2006).

41. For a literature review of body work, see Debra Gimlin, "What Is 'Body Work'? A Review of the Literature," *Sociology Compass* 1.1 (2007): 353–370.

42. Wolkowitz, *Bodies at Work*, 6.

43. E.g., Lynne Pettinger, "Gendered Work Meets Gendered Goods: Selling and Service in Clothing Retail," *Gender, Work, and Organization* 12.5 (2005): 460–478; Chris Warhurst and Dennis Nickson, "Employee Experience of Aesthetic Labour in Retail and Hospitality," *Work, Employment, and Society* 21.1 (2007): 103–120; Chris Warhurst and Dennis Nickson, "'Who's Got the Look?' Emotional, Aesthetic, and Sexualized Labour in Interactive Services," *Gender, Work, and Organization* 16.3 (2009): 385–404; Christine L. Williams and Catherine Connell, "'Looking Good and Sounding Right': Aesthetic Labor and Social Inequality in the Retail Industry," *Work and Occupations* 37.3 (2010): 349–377; Anne Witz, Chris Warhurst, and Dennis Nickson, "The Labour of Aesthetics and the Aesthetics of Organization," *Organization* 10.1 (2003): 33–54.

44. Kang, *The Managed Hand*, 13.

45. IBISWorld, *Hair and Nail Salons in the US—Industry Market Research Report* (Los Angeles: IBISWorld, August 2008); IBISWorld, *Hair and Nail Salons in the US— Industry Market Research Report* (Los Angeles: IBISWorld, August 2010).

46. Black, *The Beauty Industry*; Kang, *The Managed Hand*; Sharma and Black, "Feel Good, Look Better."

47. For a discussion of how economic change and cultural landscapes create sexualized labor, particularly in terms of prostitution but with lessons for other jobs, see Elizabeth Bernstein, *Temporarily Yours: Intimacy, Authenticity, and the Commerce of Sex* (Chicago: University of Chicago Press, 2007).

48. Ronald S. Barlow, *The Vanishing American Barbershop: An Illustrated History of Tonsorial Art 1860–1969* (St. Paul, MN: William Marvy Company, 1996); Christian R. Jones, *Barbershop: History and Antiques* (Atglen, PA: Schiffer, 1999).

49. Barber, "The Well-Coiffed Man."

50. Anne P. Crick, "Glad to Meet You—My Best Friend: Relationships in the Hospitality Industry," *Social and Economic Studies* 51.1 (2002): 99–125.

51. Michael A. Messner, *Power at Play: Sports and the Problem of Masculinity* (Boston: Beacon Press, 1992).

52. Deborah S. David and Robert Brannon, *The Forty-Nine Percent Majority: The Male Sex Role* (New York: Random House, 1976); also see Michael S. Kimmel, "Masculinity as Homophobia: Fear, Shame, and Silence in the Construction of Gender Identity," in *Theorizing Masculinities*, ed. Harry Brod and Michael Kaufman (Thousand Oaks, CA: Sage, 1994), 119–141.

53. Wade, "American Men's Hidden Crisis."

54. Eric Anderson and Mark McCormack, "Cuddling and Spooning: Heteromasculinity and Homosocial Tactility among Student-Athletes," *Men and Masculinities* 18.2 (2015): 214–230. Anderson and McCormack suggest that what I call touching rules may be shifting for men. Their research shows that young straight male British athletes enjoy cuddling and spooning with their straight male friends. Also see Mark McCormack, "Hey, Bro, Let's Cuddle: Why the Modern Man Likes to Touch," *Playboy*, August 26, 2014, http://www.playboy.com/articles/why-modern-men-like-to-cuddle.

55. Jonathon Crowe, "Men and Feminism: Some Challenges and a Partial Response," *Social Alternatives* 30.1 (2011): 49–53; Michael S. Kimmel, "'Gender Symmetry' in Domestic Violence: A Substantive and Methodological Research Review," *Violence Against Women* 8.11 (2002): 1332–1363.

CHAPTER 5 "WE'RE MEN'S WOMEN"

1. Patricia Yancey Martin, "'Said and Done' vs. 'Saying and Doing': Gendering Practices, Practicing Gender at Work," *Gender and Society* 17. 3 (2003): 342–366.

2. Candace West and Don H. Zimmerman, "Doing Gender," *Gender and Society* 1.2 (1987): 125–151. Also see Catherine Connell, "Doing, Undoing, or Redoing Gender?: Learning from the Workplace Experiences of Transpeople," *Gender and Society* 24.1 (2010): 31–55; Karen D. Pyke and Denise L. Johnson, "Asian American Women and Radicalized Femininities: 'Doing' Gender across Cultural Worlds," *Gender and Society* 17.1 (2003): 33–53; Mary Nell Trautner, "Doing Gender, Doing Class: The Performance of Sexuality in Exotic Dance Clubs," *Gender and Society* 19.6 (2005): 771–788.

3. For a discussion of young women's hierachical relationships along the lines of race, ethnicity, and class, see Julie Bettie, *Women without Class: Girls, Race, Identity* (Berkeley: University of California Press, 2003).

4. Matthew B. Ezzell, "'Barbie Dolls on the Pitch: Identity Work, Defensive Othering, and Inequality in Women's Rugby," *Social Problems* 56.1 (2009): 111. Also see Michael L. Schwalbe and Douglas Mason-Schrock, "Identity Work as Group Process," *Advance in*

Group Processes, vol. 13, ed. Shane R. Thye and Edward J. Lawler (Greenwich, CT: JAI Press, 1996), 115–149.

5. Candace West and Sarah Fenstermaker, "Doing Difference," *Gender and Society* 9.1 (1995): 8–37.

6. E.g., Paula Black, *The Beauty Industry: Gender, Culture, Pleasure* (London: Routledge, 2004); Frida Kerner Furman, *Facing the Mirror: Older Women and Beauty Shop Culture* (London: Routledge, 1997); Debra Gimlin, "Pamela's Place: Power and Negotiation in the Hair Salon," *Gender and Society* 10.5 (1996): 505–526; Lanita Jacobs-Huey, *From the Kitchen to the Parlor: Language and Becoming in African American Women's Hair Care* (New York: Oxford University Press, 2006); Kathy Peiss, *Hope in a Jar: The Making of America's Beauty Culture* (New York: Henry Holt, 1998).

7. Kris Paap, *Working Construction: Why White Working Class Men Put Themselves— and the Labor Movement—in Harm's Way* (Ithaca, NY: Cornell University Press, 2006); Jessica Smith Rolston, *Mining Coal and Undermining Gender: Rhythms of Work and Family in the American West* (New Brunswick, NJ: Rutgers University Press, 2014); Kristen Yount, "Ladies, Flirts, and Tomboys: Strategies for Managing Sexual Harassment in an Underground Coal Mine," *Journal of Contemporary Ethnography* 19.4 (1991): 396–422. Women who work with men on construction sites or in coalmines do not fit typical perceptions of women's appropriate or natural roles. Conflating masculinity with strength and technical ability makes women in such jobs both ideological and literal anomalies.

8. Chrys Ingraham, "The Heterosexual Imaginary: Feminist Sociology and Theories of Gender," *Sociological Theory* 12.2 (1994): 203–219. Ingraham's concept of the "heterosexual imaginary" captures the process of heteronormativity, especially how presumptions of heterosexuality shape cultural rituals and scholarly work. Regarding research: heterosexuality shapes what and whom scholars research, as well as how they analyze data, and silences alternative desires and relationships.

9. This is especially the case for massage parlors. See Sarah Oerton, "Bodywork Boundaries: Power, Politics, and Professionalism in Therapeutic Massage," *Gender, Work, and Organization* 11.5 (2004): 544–565; Sarah Oerton and Joanne Phoenix, "Sex/Body Work: Discourses and Practices," *Sexualities* 4.4 (2001): 387–412.

10. Research on women's relationships in beauty work and beauty consumption overlooks sexuality and thus suffers from the heterosexual imaginary. Ingraham, "The Heterosexual Imaginary."

11. Laura Rhoton, "Distancing as a Gendered Barrier: Understanding Women Scientists' Gender Practices," *Gender and Society* 25.6 (2011): 707.

12. Elin Kvande, "'In the Belly of the Beast': Constructing Femininities in Engineering Organizations," *European Journal of Women's Studies* 6.3 (1999): 309. Also see Rhoton, "Distancing as a Gendered Barrier."

13. See Sharon R. Bird and Laura A. Rhoton, "Women Professionals' Gender Strategies: Negotiating Gendered Organizational Barriers," in *Handbook of Gender, Work, and Organization*, ed. Emma Jeanas, David Knights, and Patricia Yancey Martin (Hoboken, NJ: John Wiley and Sons, 2011). 245–262; Jody Miller, *One of the Guys: Girls, Gangs, and Gender* (New York: Oxford University Press, 2001); Gillian Ranson, "No Longer 'One

of the Boys': Negotiations with Motherhood, as Prospect or Reality, among Women in Engineering," *Canadian Review of Sociology* 42.2 (2005): 145–166.

14. Michael S. Kimmel and Abby L. Ferber, eds., *Privilege* (Boulder, CO: Westview Press, 2003). Kimmel and Ferber note that middle-class white men represent the "the generic person" (3), and are considered by others to be *"unbiased,* an objective opinion—disembodied Western rationality" (4). Consider how "man," in the English language, has been considered a non-gendered descriptor used to refer to all people.

15. Ulla Forseth, "Gender Matters? Exploring How Gender Is Negotiated in Service Encounters," *Gender, Work, and Organization* 12.5 (2005): 443.

16. Rhoton, "Distancing as a Gendered Barrier," 701.

17. E.g., Patricia Hill Collins, *Black Feminist Thought: Knowledge, Consciousness, and the Politics of Empowerment* (New York: Routledge, 1990).

18. Ibid., 7.

19. For a discussion of women trading on homophobia, see Laura Hamilton, "Trading on Heterosexuality: College Women's Gender Strategies and Homophobia," *Gender and Society* 21.2 (2007): 145–172.

20. Lex Boyle, "Flexing the Tensions of Female Muscularity: How Female Bodybuilders Negotiate Normative Femininity in Competitive Bodybuilding," *Women's Studies Quarterly* 33.1–2 (2005): 134–149. Matthew B. Ezzell, "'Barbie Dolls on the Pitch: Identity Work, Defensive Othering, and Inequality in Women's Rugby," *Social Problems* 56.1 (2009): 111–131.

21. Michael S. Kimmel, "Masculinity as Homophobia: Fear, Shame, and Silence in the Construction of Gender Identity," in *Theorizing Masculinities,* ed. Harry Brod and Michael Kaufman (Thousand Oaks, CA: Sage, 1994), 125.

22. Judith Lorber, *Paradoxes of Gender* (New Haven: Yale University Press, 1994), 61.

23. Barrie Thorne, *Gender Play: Girls and Boys in School* (New Brunswick, NJ: Rutgers University Press, 1993).

24. Ibid.

25. Ariel Levy, *Female Chauvinist Pigs: Women and the Rise of Raunch Culture* (New York: Free Press, 2005).

26. Michael S. Kimmel, "Men's Responses to Feminism at the Turn of the Century," *Gender and Society* 1.3 (1987): 261–283; Michael S. Kimmel, *Manhood in America: A Cultural History* (New York: The Free Press, 1996), 16–17. Kimmel argues that contemporary meanings of manhood are tied historically to the emergence of the self-made man, who "derived identity entirely from man's activities in the public sphere, measured by accumulated wealth and status" (17). As women moved into the workforce in greater numbers, especially into previously male-dominated jobs, this caused a crisis of masculinity. Also see Messner on how a crisis in masculinity arose post-Title IX, as women flooded into sports and destabilized the idea that only men were competent athletes. Michael A. Messner, "Sports and Male Domination: The Female Athlete as Contested Ideological Terrain," *Sociology of Sport Journal* 5.3 (1988): 197–211.

27. For an exception, see Samantha A. Morgan-Curtis, "Misogyny," in *International Encyclopedia of Men and Masculinities,* ed. Michael Flood, Judith Kegan Gardiner, Bob Pease, and Keith Pringle (New York: Routledge, 2007), 443–445: "Though most common in men, misogyny also exists in and is practiced by women against other women or even themselves. Misogyny functions . . . to place women in subordinate positions [to men] with limited access to power and decision making" (443).

28. See Paula England, "Emerging Theories of Care Work," *Annual Review of Sociology* 31 (2005): 381–399; Karla A. Erickson, "To Invest or Detach? Coping Strategies and Workplace Culture in Service Work," *Symbolic Interaction* 27.4 (2004): 549–572; Carla Freeman, *High Tech and High Heels in the Global Economy: Women, Work, and Pink-Collar Identities in the Caribbean* (Durham, NC: Duke University Press, 2000); Arlie Hochschild, *The Managed Heart: Commercialization of Human Feeling* (Berkeley: University of California Press, 1983); Lynn May Rivas, "Invisible Labors: Caring for the Independent Person," in *Global Woman: Nannies, Maids, and Sex Workers in the New Economy*, ed. Barbara Ehrenreich and Arlie Russell Hochschild (New York: Henry Holt and Company, 2002), 70–84.

29. Yvonne A. Tamayo, "Rhymes with Rich: Power, Law, and the Bitch," *St. Thomas Law Review* 21.3 (2009): 281–301.

30. American Association of University Women (AAUW), "The Simple Truth about the Gender Pay Gap," (Washington, DC: AAUW, 2014), http://www.aauw.org/files/2014/03/The-Simple-Truth.pdf; Michelle J. Budig and Melissa J. Hodges, "Differences in Disadvantage: Variations in the Motherhood Penalty Across White Women's Earnings Distributions," *American Sociological Review* 75.5 (2010): 705–728; Philip N. Cohen and Matt L. Huffman, "Individuals, Jobs, and Labor Markets: The Devaluation of Women's Work," *American Sociological Review* 68.3 (2003): 443–463; Francine D. Blau and Lawrence M. Kahn, "The Gender Pay Gap: Have Women Gone as Far as They Can?" *Academy of Management Perspectives* 21.1 (2007): 7–23.

31. See Sharon Hays, *The Cultural Contradictions of Motherhood* (New Haven, CT: Yale University Press, 1996); Pamela Stone, *Opting Out?: Why Women Really Quit Careers and Head Home* (Berkeley: University of California Press, 2007).

32. Kristen Barber, "The Well-Coiffed Man: Class, Race, and Heterosexual Masculinity in the Hair Salon," *Gender and Society* 22.4 (2008): 455–476; Kristen Barber, "Styled Masculinity: Men's Consumption of Salon Hair Care and the Construction of Difference," in *Exploring Masculinities: Identity, Inequality, Continuity and Change*, ed. C. J. Pascoe and Tristan Bridges (Oxford: Oxford University Press, 2015), 69–79.

33. Anne Fausto-Sterling, *Myths of Gender: Biological Theories about Women and Men* (1985; rpt. New York: Basic Books, 1992); Anne Fausto-Sterling, *Sexing the Body: Gender Politics and the Construction of Sexuality* (New York: Basic Books, 2000). Also see Daniel J. Moskovic, Michael L. Eisenberg, and Larry I. Lipshultz, "Seasonal Fluctuations in Testosterone-Estrogen Ratio in Men from the Southwest United States," *Journal of Andrology* 33.6 (2012): 1298–1304; Women's Health Program, Women's Health Program, Monash University, "Testosterone and Androgens in Women," October 2010, http://med.monash.edu.au/sphspm/womenshealth/docs/testosterone-and-androgens-in-women.pdf.

34. Laura Briggs, "The Race of Hysteria: 'Overcivilization' and the 'Savage' Woman in Late Nineteenth-Century Obstetrics and Gynecology," *American Quarterly* 52.2 (2000):

246–273; Rachel P. Maines, *The Technology of Orgasm: "Hysteria," the Vibrator, and Women's Sexual Satisfaction* (Baltimore, MD: Johns Hopkins University Press, 1998).

35. Maines, *The Technology of Orgasm*. Nineteenth-century gynecologists and psychotherapists declared women vulnerable to their uteruses, which supposedly wandered around women's bodies creating numerous ailments. This Cartesian mind-body dualism reduced women to their reproductive biology and exalted men as rational beings ripe for powerful, public, decision-making roles. The cure for female hysteria, caused by a wandering uterus or sexual repression, was a pelvic massage by a male physician to the point of "hysterical paroxysm" (3). Physicians often found this treatment tiring and difficult to accomplish, and so would refer afflicted women to the care of midwives.

36. Anne Fausto-Sterling, "The Five Sexes: Why Male and Female Are Not Enough," *The Sciences* 33.2 (1993): 20–24; Judith Lorber, "Beyond the Binaries: Depolarizing the Categories of Sex, Sexuality, and Gender," *Sociological Inquiry* 66.2 (1996): 143–160; Judith Lorber, *Breaking the Bowls: Degendering and Feminist Change* (New York: W. W. Norton, 2005); Mimi Schippers, "Recovering the Feminine Other: Masculinity, Femininity, and Gender Hegemony," *Theory and Society* 36.1 (2007): 85–102.

37. Peiss, *Hope in a Jar.*

38. For a discussion of women jockeying for the role of beauty expert, see Gimlin, "Pamela's Place."

39. Adia Harvey Wingfield, *Doing Business with Beauty: Black Women, Hair Salons, and the Racial Enclave Economy* (New York: Rowman and Littlefield, 2008); Julia A. Willett, *Permanent Waves: The Making of the American Beauty Shop* (New York: New York University Press, 2000).

40. Barber, "The Well-Coiffed Man"; Barber, "Styled Masculinity."

41. See Gimlin, "Pamela's Place."

42. Schippers, "Recovering the Feminine Other."

43. Raewyn Connell, *Gender and Power* (Stanford, CA: Stanford University Press, 1987).

44. Schippers, "Recovering the Feminine Other."

45. Ibid., 86. Also see Judith Halberstam, *Female Masculinity* (Durham, NC: Duke University Press, 1998).

46. Bird and Rhoton, "Women Professionals' Gender Strategies"; Miller, *One of the Guys*; Ranson, "No Longer 'One of the Boys.'"

47. West and Fenstermaker, "Doing Difference."

CONCLUSION

1. "George Clooney Is Voted the Top Silver Fox: Actor Beats Brad Pitt and Johnny Depp to Win Man Ageing Gracefully Poll," *Daily Mail*, August 31, 2014, http://www.dailymail.co.uk/news/article-2739175/Clooney-voted-silver-fox-Actor-beats-Brad-Pitt-Johnny-Depp-win-Man-Ageing-Gracefully-poll.html.

2. Lynne Luciano, *Looking Good: Male Body Image in Modern America* (New York: Hill and Wang, 2001).

3. Susan Campos, "Leg Hair Transplants and Scalp Tattoos: How Hollywood's A-List Fights Baldness," *Hollywood Reporter*, October 3, 2013, http://www.hollywoodreporter .com/news/leg-hair-transplants-scalp-tattoos-639796.

4. "George Clooney Travels with His Own Hair Stylist! (Who's a Pretty Boy?)" *VH1* online video, December 5, 2013, http://www.vh1.com/video/misc/984645/george -clooney-travels-with-his-own-hair-stylist-whos-a-pretty-boy.jhtml.

5. See Kristen Barber, "The Well-Coiffed Man: Class, Race, and Heterosexual Masculinity in the Hair Salon," *Gender and Society* 22.4 (2008): 455–476; Kristen Barber, "Styled Masculinity: Men's Consumption of Salon Hair Care and the Construction of Difference," in *Exploring Masculinities: Identity, Inequality, Continuity and Change*, ed. C. J. Pascoe and Tristan Bridges. (Cambridge, U.K.: Oxford University Press, 2015), 69–79.

6. Fabio Musso and Elena Druica, *Handbook of Research on Retailer-Consumer Relationship Development* (Hershey, PA: IGI Global, 2014), 126.

7. Nick Crossley, "Merleau-Ponty, the Elusive Body, and Carnal Sociology," *Body & Society* 1.1 (1995): 48.

8. Michel Foucault, "Body/Power," in *Power/Knowledge: Selected Interviews and Other Writings 1972–1977*, ed. Colin Gordon (New York: Pantheon Books, 1975), 55.

9. See Jean Baudrillard, *The Consumer Society: Myths and Structures* (Thousand Oaks, CA: Sage Publications, 1998).

10. Euromonitor International, *Men's Grooming Products—US* (London: Euromonitor International, May 2008); IBISWorld, *Hair and Nail Salons in the US—Industry Market Research Report* (Los Angeles: IBISWorld, August 2008).

11. Michael Quintanilla, "H-E-B Aisle Is for Guys Only," *Houston Chronicle*, January 27, 2010, http://www.chron.com/life/article/H-E-B-aisle-is-for-guys-only-1708148.php.

12. C. J. Pascoe, *Dude, You're a Fag: Masculinity and Sexuality in High School* (Berkeley: University of California Press, 2007), 183.

13. E.g., Debra Gimlin, "Pamela's Place: Power and Negotiation in the Hair Salon," *Gender and Society* 10.5 (1996): 505–526.

14. Candace West and Sarah Fenstermaker, "Doing Difference," *Gender and Society* 9.1 (1995): 8–37.

15. Louis Williams, "The Relationship between a Black Barbershop and the Community That Supports It," *Human Mosaic* 27.1–2 (1993): 29–33; Earl Wright II, "More Than Just a Haircut: Sociability within the Urban African American Barbershop," *Challenge: A Journal of Research on African American Men* 9 (1998): 1–13; Earl Wright II and Thomas C. Calhoun, "From the Common Thug to the Local Businessman: An Exploration into an Urban African American Barbershop," *Deviant Behavior: An Interdisciplinary Journal* 22.3 (2001): 267–288.

16. E.g., Rose Weitz, *Rapunzel's Daughters: What Women's Hair Tells Us about Women's Lives* (New York: Farrar, Straus and Giroux, 2004).

17. Gimlin, "Pamela's Place."

18. Shari L. Dworkin and Michael A. Messner, "Just Do . . . What?: Sports, Bodies, Gender," in *Revisioning Gender*, ed. Myra Marx Ferree, Judith Lorber, and Beth B. Hess (Lanham, MD: AltaMira Press, 1999), 341–361; Michael A. Messner, "Barbie Girls

versus Sea Monsters: Children Constructing Gender," *Gender and Society* 14.6 (2000): 765–784.

19. Miliann Kang, "The Managed Hand: The Commercialization of Bodies and Emotions in Korean Immigrant-Owned Nail Salons," *Gender and Society* 17.6 (2003): 820–839; Miliann Kang, *The Managed Hand: Race, Gender, and the Body in Beauty Service Work* (Berkeley: University of California Press, 2010).

20. Rachel Sherman, *Class Acts: Service and Inequality in Luxury Hotels* (Berkeley: University of California Press, 2007).

21. Kang, "The Managed Hand"; Kang, *The Managed Hand*.

22. Julia A. Willett, *Permanent Waves: The Making of the American Beauty Shop* (New York: New York University Press, 2000).

23. Monica Davey, "Wisconsin Justices Uphold Union Limits, a Victory for the Governor," *New York Times*, July 31, 2007, http://www.nytimes.com/2014/08/01/us/wisconsin-union-limits-and-voter-id-law-upheld-by-court.html?_r=0.

24. Michael A. Fletcher, "Fast-Food Workers Plan a New Wave of Walkouts across the Nation," *Washington Post*, December 3, 2013, http://www.washingtonpost.com/business/economy/fast-food-workers-plan-a-new-wave-of-walkouts-across-the-nation/2013/12/03/b64809e4-5b87-11e3-a49b-90a0e156254b_story.html.

APPENDIX A

1. See the Economic Policy Institute, "The Great Recession," 2014, http://stateof workingamerica.org/great-recession/.

2. The 2009 unemployment rate in the Los Angeles area was as high as 11.6 in July. U.S. Department of Labor, Bureau of Labor Statistics, "Household Data Annual Averages: Employed Status of the Civilian Noninstitutional Population, 1944 to Date" (Washington, DC: Bureau of Labor Statistics, 2015); U.S. Department of Labor, Bureau of Labor Statistics, "Databases, Tables, & Calculators by Subject: Los Angeles–Long Beach–Anaheim, CA Metropolitan Statistical Area Unemployment Rate" (Washington, DC: Bureau of Labor Statistics, 2015).

3. Greg Burns, "Evidence Shows There's No Such Thing as 'Recession-Proof Jobs," *Chicago Tribune*, July 20, 2009, http://articles.chicagotribune.com/2009-07-20/news/0907190129_1_recession-proof-bankruptcy-lawyers-william-hummer.

4. Market research on U.S. hair and nail salons supports the assumption that "when unemployment increases, clients are less likely to indulge in higher value salon services." IBISWorld, *Hair and Nail Salons in the US—IBISWorld Industry Report 81211* (Los Angeles: IBISWorld, February 2015), 6.

5. See Ronald E. Hallett and Kristen Barber, "Ethnographic Research in a Cyber Era," *Journal of Contemporary Ethnography* 43.3 (2014): 306–330.

6. Joseph A. Conti and Moira O'Neil, "Studying Power: Qualitative Methods and Global Elite," *Qualitative Research* 7.1 (2007): 63–82.

7. Kristen Barber, "Studying Men and Beauty: The Masculinity Challenge and Cross-Gender Research as an Opportunity for Redemption," in progress.

8. See Annette Lareau, *Unequal Childhoods: Class, Race, and Family Life* (Berkeley: University of California Press, 2003).

9. Neil Stephens, "Collecting Data from Elites and Ultra Elites: Telephone and Face-to-Face Interviews with Macroeconomists," *Qualitative Research* 7.2 (2007): 203–216.

10. For a discussion of researcher's gender in the in-depth interview, see Christine L. Williams and E. Joel Heikes, "The Importance of Researcher's Gender in the In-Depth Interview: Evidence from Two Case Studies of Male Nurses," *Gender and Society* 7.2 (1993): 280–291.

11. See Barber, "Studying Men and Beauty."

12. Terry Arendell, "Reflections on the Researcher-Researched Relationship: A Woman Interviewing Men," *Qualitative Sociology* 20.3 (1997): 341–368; Caroline Gatrell, "Interviewing Fathers: Feminist Dilemmas in Fieldwork," *Journal of Gender Studies* 15.3 (2006): 237–257; Barry Levinson, "(How) Can a Man Do Feminist Ethnography of Education?" *Qualitative Inquiry* 4.3 (1998): 337–369; Lois Presser, "Negotiating Power and Narrative in Research: Implications for Feminist Methodology," *Signs: Journal of Women in Culture and Society* 30.4 (2005): 2067–2090; Rosaline H. Wax, "Gender and Age in Fieldwork and Fieldwork Education: 'Not Any Good Thing Is Done by One Man Alone,'" in *Self, Sex, and Gender in Cross-Cultural Fieldwork*, ed. Tony L. Whitehead and Mary E. Conaway (1970, Reprint. Chicago: University of Illinois Press, 1986), 129–150.

13. Michael L. Schwalbe and Michelle Wolkomir, "The Masculine Self as Problem and Resource in Interview Studies of Men," *Men and Masculinities* 4.1 (2001): 93.

14. Verta Taylor and Leila J. Rupp, "When the Girls Are Men: Negotiating Gender and Sexual Dynamics in a Study of Drag Queens," *Signs: Journal of Women in Culture and Society* 30.4 (2005): 2115–2139.

15. Patricia Hill Collins, *Black Feminist Thought: Knowledge, Consciousness, and the Politics of Empowerment* (New York: Routledge, 1990); Sharlene Nagy Hesse-Biber and Michelle L. Yaiser, eds., *Feminist Perspectives on Social Research* (Oxford: Oxford University Press, 2004); Liz Stanley and Sue Wise, *Breaking Out: Feminist Consciousness and Feminist Research* (London: Routledge and Kegan Paul, 1983).

16. Mary Dankoski, "What Makes Research Feminist?" *Journal of Feminist Family Therapy* 12.1 (2000): 3–19; Ann Oakley, "Interviewing Women: A Contradiction in Terms?" in *Doing Feminist Research*, ed. Helen Roberts (London: Routledge and Kegan Paul, 1981), 30–61; Judith Stacey, "Can There Be a Feminist Ethnography?" *Women's Studies International Forum* 11.1 (1988): 21–27; Diane L. Wolf, "Situating Feminist Dilemmas in Fieldwork," in *Feminist Dilemmas in Fieldwork*, ed. Diane L. Wolf (Boulder, CO: Westview Press, 1996), 1–55.

17. James W. Messerschmidt, *Nine Lives: Adolescent Masculinities, the Body, and Violence* (Boulder, CO: Westview Press, 2000); James W. Messerschmidt, "Becoming 'Real Men': Adolescent Masculinity Challenges and Sexual Violence," *Men and Masculinities* 2.3 (2000): 286–307.

18. Barber, "Studying Men and Beauty."

BIBLIOGRAPHY

Acker, Joan. "Hierarchies, Jobs, Bodies: A Theory of Gendered Organizations." *Gender and Society* 4.2 (1990): 139–158.

———. "Inequality Regimes: Gender, Class, and Race in Organizations." *Gender and Society* 20.4 (2006): 441–464.

Adkins, Lisa. "Mobile Desire: Aesthetics, Sexuality, and the 'Lesbian' at Work." *Sexualities* 3.2 (2000): 201–218.

Alexander, Bryant K. "Fading, Twisting, and Weaving: An Interpretive Ethnography of the Black Barbershop as Cultural Space." *Qualitative Inquiry* 9.1 (2003): 105–128.

———. *Performing Black Masculinity: Race, Culture, and Queer Identity.* Lanham, MD: AltaMira Press, 2006.

Alexander, Susan M. "Stylish Hard Bodies: Masculinity in Men's Health Magazines." *Sociological Perspectives* 46.4 (2003): 535–554.

Allison, Anne. *Nightwork: Sexuality, Pleasure, and Corporate Masculinity in a Tokyo Hostess Club.* Chicago: University of Chicago Press, 1994.

Alvarez, Luis. *The Power of the Zoot: Youth Culture and Resistance during World War II.* Berkeley: University of California Press, 2009.

American Association of University Women (AAUW). "The Simple Truth about the Gender Pay Gap." Washington, DC: AAUW, 2014. http://www.aauw.org/files/2014/03/The-Simple-Truth.pdf.

Anderson, Eric, and Mark McCormack. "Cuddling and Spooning: Heteromasculinity and Homosocial Tactility among Student-Athletes." *Men and Masculinities* 18.2 (2015): 214–230.

Arendell, Terry. "Reflections on the Researcher-Researched Relationship: A Woman Interviewing Men." *Qualitative Sociology* 20.3 (1997): 341–368.

Barber, Kristen. "Studying Men and Beauty: The Masculinity Challenge and Cross-Gender Research as an Opportunity for Redemption." In progress.

———. "Styled Masculinity: Men's Consumption of Salon Hair Care and the Construction of Difference." In *Exploring Masculinities: Identity, Inequality, Continuity, and Change,* edited by C. J. Pascoe and Tristan Bridges, 69–79. Oxford: Oxford University Press, 2015.

———. "The Well-Coiffed Man: Class, Race, and Heterosexual Masculinity in the Hair Salon." *Gender and Society* 22.4 (2008): 455–476.

Barlow, Ronald S. *The Vanishing American Barbershop: An Illustrated History of Tonsorial Art 1860–1969.* St. Paul, MN: William Marvy Company, 1996.

Bates, Timothy, William E. Jackson III, and James H. Johnson Jr. "Introduction: Advancing Research on Minority Entrepreneurship." *Annals of the American Academy of Political and Social Science* 613 (2007): 10–17.

Battle-Walters, Kimberly. *Sheila's Shop: Working Class African American Women Talk about Life, Love, Race, and Hair*. Lanham, MD: Rowman & Littlefield, 2004.

Baudrillard, Jean. *The Consumer Society: Myths and Structures*. Thousand Oaks, CA: Sage Publications, 1998.

Baumgardner, Jennifer, and Amy Richards. "Who's the Next Gloria? The Quest for the Third Wave Superleader." In *Catching a Wave: Reclaiming Feminism for the 21st Century*, edited by Rory Dicker and Alison Piepmeier, 159–170. Boston: Northeastern University Press, 2003.

Bernstein, Elizabeth. *Temporarily Yours: Intimacy, Authenticity, and the Commerce of Sex*. Chicago: University of Chicago Press, 2007.

Bettie, Julie. *Women without Class: Girls, Race, Identity*. Berkeley: University of California Press, 2003.

Bianchi, Suzanne M., Liana C. Sayer, Melissa A. Milkie, and John P. Robinson. "Housework: Who Did, Does or Will Do It, and How Much Does it Matter?" *Social Forces* 91.1 (2012): 55–63.

Bird, Sharon R. "Welcome to the Men's Club: Homosociability and the Maintenance of Hegemonic Masculinity." *Gender and Society* 10.2 (1996): 120–132.

Bird, Sharon R., and Laura A. Rhoton. "Women Professionals' Gender Strategies: Negotiating Gendered Organizational Barriers." In *Handbook of Gender, Work, and Organization*, edited by Emma Jeanas, David Knights, and Patricia Yancey Martin, 245–262. Hoboken, NJ: John Wiley and Sons, 2011.

Black, Paula. *The Beauty Industry: Gender, Culture, Pleasure*. London: Routledge, 2004.

———. "'Ordinary People Come Through Here': Locating the Beauty Salon in Women's Lives." *Feminist Review* 71.1 (2002): 2–17.

Blau, Francine D., and Lawrence M. Kahn. "The Gender Pay Gap: Have Women Gone as Far as They Can?" *Academy of Management Perspectives* 21.1 (2007): 7–23.

Blickenstaff, Jacob Clark. "Women and Science Careers: Leaky Pipeline or Gender Filter?" *Gender and Education* 17.4 (2005): 369–386.

Bordo, Susan. *The Male Body: A New Look at Men in Public and in Private*. New York: Farrar, Straus, and Giroux, 1999.

Bourdieu, Pierre. *Distinction: A Social Critique of the Judgment of Taste*. Cambridge, MA: Harvard University Press, 1984.

Boyd, Robert L. "Depletion of the South's Human Capital: The Case of Eminent Black Entrepreneurs." *Southeastern Geographer* 49.3 (2009): 251–266.

———. "Transformation of the Black Business Elite." *Social Science Quarterly* 87.3 (2006): 602–617.

Boyle, Lex. "Flexing the Tensions of Female Muscularity: How Female Bodybuilders Negotiate Normative Femininity in Competitive Bodybuilding." *Women's Studies Quarterly* 33.1–2 (2005): 134–149.

Brandon, Ruth. *Ugly Beauty: Helena Rubinstein, L'Oréal, and the Blemished History of Looking Good*. New York: HarperCollins, 2011.

Brannick, Teresa, and David Coghlan. "In Defense of Being 'Native': The Case for Insider Academic Research." *Organisational Research Methods* 10.1 (2007): 59–74.

Breazeale, Kenon. "In Spite of Women: *Esquire* Magazine and the Construction of the Male Consumer." In *The Gender and Consumer Culture Reader*, edited by Jennifer Scanlon, 226–244. New York: New York University Press, 2000.

Bridges, Tristan. "Bacon, Beards, and Beer: Feminist Reflections on Hipster Masculinity." *The Society Pages*, July 31, 2014. http://thesocietypages.org/feminist/2014/07/31/bacon-beards-and-beer-feminist-reflections-on-hipster-masculinity.

———. "Gender Capital and Male Bodybuilders." *Body and Society* 15.1 (2009): 83–107.

———. "A Very 'Gay' Straight? Hybrid Masculinities, Sexual Aesthetics, and the Changing Relationship between Masculinity and Homophobia." *Gender and Society* 28.1 (2014): 58–82.

Bridges, Tristan, and C. J. Pascoe. "Hybrid Masculinities: New Directions in the Sociology of Men and Masculinities." *Sociology Compass* 8.3 (2014): 246–258.

Briggs, Laura. "The Race of Hysteria: 'Overcivilization' and the 'Savage' Woman in Late Nineteenth-Century Obstetrics and Gynecology." *American Quarterly* 52.2 (2000): 246–273.

Britton, Dana M. "The Epistemology of the Gendered Organization." *Gender and Society* 14.3 (2000): 418–434.

Budig, Michelle J., and Melissa J. Hodges. "Differences in Disadvantage: Variations in the Motherhood Penalty Across White Women's Earnings Distributions." *American Sociological Review* 75.5 (2010): 705–728.

Bulan, Heather Ferguson, Rebecca J. Erickson, and Amy S. Wharton. "Doing for Others on the Job: The Affective Requirements of Service Work, Gender, and Emotional Well-Being." *Social Problems* 44.2 (1997): 235–256.

Burleson, Brant R. "A Different Voice on Different Cultures: Illusion and Reality in the Study of Sex Differences in Personal Relationships." *Personal Relationships* 4.3 (2005): 229–241.

Burns, Greg. "Evidence Shows There's No Such Thing as 'Recession-Proof' Jobs." *Chicago Tribune*, July 20, 2009. http://articles.chicagotribune.com/2009–07–20/news/0907190129_1_recession-proof-bankruptcy-lawyers-william-hummer.

Butler, Judith. *Gender Trouble: Feminism and the Subversion of Identity*. New York: Routledge, Chapman & Hall, 1990.

Campos, Susan. "Leg Hair Transplants and Scalp Tattoos: How Hollywood's A-List Fights Baldness." *Hollywood Reporter*, October 3, 2013. http://www.hollywoodreporter.com/news/leg-hair-transplants-scalp-tattoos-639796.

Cashmore, Ellis. "David Beckham: Rise of the Metrosexual." *CNN*. Last modified May 17, 2013. http://www.cnn.com/2013/05/17/opinion/beckham-metro-symbol/.

Chauncey, George. *Gay New York: Gender, Urban Culture, and the Making of the Gay Male World, 1890–1940*. New York: Basic Books, 1995.

Chesley, Noelle. "Stay-at-Home Fathers and Breadwinning Mothers: Gender, Couple Dynamics, and Social Change." *Gender and Society* 25.5 (2011): 642–664.

Coad, David. *The Metrosexual: Gender, Sexuality, and Sports*. Albany: State University of New York Press, 2008.

Cogan, Jeanine C. "Lesbians Walk the Tightrope of Beauty: Thin Is In but Femme Is Out." *Journal of Lesbian Studies* 3.4 (1999): 77–89.

Cohen, Philip N., and Matt L. Huffman. "Individuals, Jobs, and Labor Markets: The Devaluation of Women's Work." *American Sociological Review* 68.3 (2003): 443–463.

Collins, Patricia Hill. *Black Feminist Thought: Knowledge, Consciousness, and the Politics of Empowerment.* New York: Routledge, 1990.

———. "Learning from the Outsider Within: The Sociological Significance of Black Feminist Thought." *Social Problems* 33.6 (1986): 14–19.

———. "Transforming the Inner Circle: Dorothy Smith's Challenge to Sociological Theory." *Sociological Theory* 10.1 (1992): 73–80.

Coltrane, Scott. "Research on Household Labor: Modeling and Measuring the Social Embeddedness of Routine Family Work." *Journal of Marriage and Family* 62.4 (2000): 1208–1233.

Condé Nast. New York: Condé Nast. Accessed 12/10/2015. http://www.condenast .com/brands/gq/media-kit/print.

Connell, Catherine. "Doing, Undoing, or Redoing Gender?: Learning from the Workplace Experiences of Transpeople." *Gender and Society* 24.1 (2010): 31–55.

Connell, Raewyn. *Gender.* Cambridge: Polity Press, 2002.

———. *Gender and Power.* Stanford, CA: Stanford University Press, 1987.

———. *Masculinities.* Berkeley: University of California Press, 1995.

Conti, Joseph A., and Moira O'Neil. "Studying Power: Qualitative Methods and Global Elite." *Qualitative Research* 7.1 (2007): 63–82.

Cotterill, Pamela. "Interviewing Women: Issues of Friendship, Vulnerability, and Power." *Women's Studies International Forum* 15.5 (1992): 593–606.

Craig, Maxine Leeds. "Race, Beauty, and the Tangled Knot of Guilty Pleasure." *Feminist Theory* 7.2 (2006): 159–177.

Craig, Maxine Leeds, and Rita Liberti. "'Cause That's What Girls Do': The Making of a Feminized Gym." *Gender and Society* 21.5 (2007): 676–699.

Crick, Anne P. "Glad to Meet You—My Best Friend: Relationships in the Hospitality Industry." *Social and Economic Studies* 51.1 (2002): 99–125.

Crossley, Nick. "Merleau-Ponty, the Elusive Body and Carnal Sociology." *Body & Society* 1.1 (1995): 43–63.

Crowe, Jonathon. "Men and Feminism: Some Challenges and a Partial Response." *Social Alternatives* 30.1 (2011): 49–53.

Dankoski, Mary. "What Makes Research Feminist?" *Journal of Feminist Family Therapy* 12.1 (2000): 3–19.

Davey, Monica. "Wisconsin Justices Uphold Union Limits, a Victory for the Governor." *New York Times,* July 31, 2014. http://www.nytimes.com/2014/08/01/us/ wisconsin-union-limits-and-voter-id-law-upheld-by-court.html?_r=0.

David, Deborah S., and Robert Brannon. *The Forty-Nine Percent Majority: The Male Sex Role.* New York: Random House, 1976.

Dellinger, Kristen, and Christine L. Williams. "The Locker Room and the Dorm Room: Workplace Norms and Magazine Editing." *Social Problems* 49.2 (2002): 242–257.

———. "Make-Up at Work: Negotiating Appearance Rules in the Workplace." *Gender and Society* 11.2 (1997): 151–177.

Demetriou, Demetrakis Z. "Connell's Concept of Hegemonic Masculinity: A Critique." *Theory and Society* 30.3 (2001): 337–361.

Denissen, Amy M. "Crossing the Line: How Women in the Building Trades Interpret and Respond to Sexual Conduct at Work." *Journal of Contemporary Ethnography* 39.3 (2010): 297–327.

Doll, Jen. "New 'Retrosexuals' Really Just Metrosexuals with a Wardrobe Change." *The Village Voice Blogs*, April 7, 2010. http://www.villagevoice.com/news/new-retrosexuals-really-just-metrosexuals-with-a-wardrobe-change-6711384.

Du Bois, W.E.B. "The Twelfth Census and the Negro Problems." *The Southern Workman* 29.5 (1900): 305–309.

Duncan, Margaret Carlisle. "The Politics of Women's Body Images and Practices: Foucault, the Panopticon, and *Shape* Magazine." *Journal of Sport and Social Issues* 18.1 (1994): 48–65.

Dworkin, Shari L., and Michael A. Messner. "Just Do . . . What?: Sports, Bodies, Gender." In *Revisioning Gender*, edited by Myra Marx Ferree, Judith Lorber, and Beth B. Hess, 341–361. Lanham, MD: AltaMira Press, 1999.

Economic Policy Institute. "The Great Recession." http://stateofworkingamerica.org/great-recession/, 2014.

Ehrenreich, Barbara, and Arlie Russell Hochschild, eds. *Global Woman: Nannies, Maids, and Sex Workers in the New Economy.* New York: Henry Holt and Company, 2004.

England, Paula. "Emerging Theories of Care Work." *Annual Review of Sociology* 31 (2005): 381–399.

Entwistle, Joanne. *The Fashioned Body: Fashion, Dress and Modern Social Theory.* Cambridge: Polity, 2000.

Erickson, Karla A. *The Hungry Cowboy: Service and Community in a Neighborhood Restaurant.* Jackson: University Press of Mississippi, 2009.

———. "To Invest or Detach? Coping Strategies and Workplace Culture in Service Work." *Symbolic Interaction* 27.4 (2004): 549–572.

Erickson, Karla A., and Jennifer L. Pierce. "Farewell to the Organization Man: The Feminization of Loyalty in High-End and Low-End Service Jobs." *Ethnography* 6.3 (2005): 283–313.

Euromonitor International. *Men's Grooming Products—US.* London: Euromonitor International, May 2008.

———. *Men's Grooming Products—US.* London: Euromonitor International, May 2010.

———. *Men's Grooming in the US.* London: Euromonitor International, May 2015.

Ezzell, Matthew B. "'Barbie Dolls on the Pitch: Identity Work, Defensive Othering, and Inequality in Women's Rugby." *Social Problems* 56.1 (2009): 111–131.

Fausto-Sterling, Anne. "The Five Sexes: Why Male and Female Are Not Enough." *The Sciences* 33.2 (1993): 20–24.

———. *Myths of Gender: Biological Theories about Women and Men.* 1985. Reprint. New York: Basic Books, 1992.

———. *Sexing the Body: Gender Politics and the Construction of Sexuality*. New York: Basic Books, 2000.

Fletcher, Michael A. "Fast-Food Workers Plan a New Wave of Walkouts across the Nation." *Washington Post*, December 3, 2013. http://www.washingtonpost.com/business/economy/fast-food-workers-plan-a-new-wave-of-walkouts-across-the-nation/2013/12/03/b64809e4–5b87–11e3-a49b-90a0e156254b_story.html.

Flügel, John C. *The Psychology of Clothes*. London: Hogarth Press, 1930.

Forseth, Ulla. "Gender Matters? Exploring How Gender is Negotiated in Service Encounters." *Gender, Work, and Organization* 12.5 (2005): 440–459.

Foucault, Michel. "Body/Power." In *Power/Knowledge: Selected Interviews and Other Writings 1972–1977*, edited by Colin Gordon, 55–62. New York: Pantheon Books, 1975.

———. *Discipline and Punish: The Birth of the Prison*. New York: Pantheon Books, 1975.

Franklin, Clyde W. II. "The Black Male Urban Barbershop as a Sex-Role Socialization Setting." *Sex Roles* 12.9–10 (1985): 965–979.

Freeman, Carla. *High Tech and High Heels in the Global Economy: Women, Work, and Pink-Collar Identities in the Caribbean*. Durham, NC: Duke University Press, 2000.

Furman, Frida Kerner. *Facing the Mirror: Older Women and Beauty Shop Culture*. London: Routledge, 1997.

Garfinkel, Harold. *Studies in Ethnomethodology*. Englewood Cliffs, NJ: Prentice-Hall, 1967.

Gatrell, Caroline. "Interviewing Fathers: Feminist Dilemmas in Fieldwork." *Journal of Gender Studies* 15.3 (2006): 237–257.

Gentleman's Quarterly. "Armpit Hair: To Shave or Not to Shave?," *GQ*, October 14, 2000, http://www.gq.com/style/style-guy/grooming/200010/shave-armpits.

———. "The Man Bag Mans Up," *GQ*, October 2010, http://www.gq.com/style/wear-it-now/201010/man-bags-purse-briefcase-satchel-messenger-bag#slide=1.

———. "The New Business Casual," *GQ*, September 2010, http://www.gq.com/style/wear-it-now/201009/new-business-casual-september-gq-style#slide=1.

———. "Pomade and the Slicked-Back Look," *GQ*, May 14, 2001, http://www.gq.com/style/style-guy/grooming/200105/slicked-back-pat-riley-ed-burns.

George, Molly. "Interactions in Expert Service Work: Demonstrating Professionalism in Personal Training." *Journal of Contemporary Ethnography* 37.1 (2008): 108–131.

"George Clooney Is Voted the Top Silver Fox: Actor Beats Brad Pitt and Johnny Depp to Win Man Ageing Gracefully Poll." Daily Mail, August 31, 2014. http://www.dailymail.co.uk/news/article-2739175/Clooney-voted-silver-fox-Actor-beats-Brad-Pitt-Johnny-Depp-win-Man-Ageing-Gracefully-poll.html.

"George Clooney Travels with His Own Hair Stylist! (Who's a Pretty Boy?)" *VH1* online video, 3:00. December 5, 2013. http://www.vh1.com/video/misc/984645/george-clooney-travels-with-his-own-hair-stylist-whos-a-pretty-boy.jhtml.

Germov, John, and Lauren Williams. "Dieting Women: Self-Surveillance and the Body Panopticon." In *Weighty Issues: Fatness and Thinness as Social Problems*, edited by Jeffry Sobal and Donna Maurer, 117–132. Hawthorne, NY: Aldine, 1999.

Gimlin, Debra. "Pamela's Place: Power and Negotiation in the Hair Salon." *Gender and Society* 10.5 (1996): 505–526.

———. "What Is 'Body Work'? A Review of the Literature." *Sociology Compass* 1.1 (2007): 353–370.

Giuffre, Patti A., and Christine L. Williams. "Boundary Lines: Labeling Sexual Harassment in Restaurants." *Gender and Society* 8.3 (1994): 378–401.

Giuffre, Patti A., Kirsten Dellinger, and Christine L. Williams. "No Retribution for Being Gay?: Inequality in Gay-Friendly Workplaces." *Sociological Spectrum* 28.3 (2008): 254–277.

Goffman, Erving. "On Face-Work: An Analysis of Ritual Elements of Social Interaction." *Psychiatry: Journal for the Study of Interpersonal Processes* 18.3 (1955): 213–231.

Goldhill, Simon. *Love, Sex, and Tragedy: How the Ancient World Shapes Our Lives.* Chicago: University of Chicago Press, 2004.

Gramsci, Antonio. *Selections from the Prison Notebooks,* edited by Quintin Hoare and Geoffrey Nowell Smith. New York: International Publishers, 1971.

Greif, Geoffrey. *Buddy System: Understanding Male Friendships.* Oxford: Oxford University Press, 2008.

Gruys, Kjerstin. "Does This Make Me Look Fat?: Aesthetic Labor and Fat Talk as Emotional Labor in a Women's Plus-Size Clothing Store." *Social Problems* 59.4 (2012): 481–500.

Gunderson, Erik. *Staging Masculinity: The Rhetoric of Performance in the Roman World.* Ann Arbor: University of Michigan Press, 2000.

Gutek, Barbara A., Charles Y. Nakamura, Martin Gahart, Inger Handschumacher, and Dan Russell. "Sexuality and the Workplace." *Basic and Applied Social Psychology* 1.3 (1980): 255–265.

Halberstam, Judith. *Female Masculinity.* Durham, NC: Duke University Press, 1998.

Hall, Jeffrey A. "Sex Differences in Friendship Expectations: A Meta-Analysis." *Journal of Social and Personal Relationships* 28.6 (2011): 723–747.

Hallett, Ronald E., and Kristen Barber. "Ethnographic Research in a Cyber Era." *Journal of Contemporary Ethnography* 43.3 (2014): 306–330.

Hamilton, Laura. "Trading on Heterosexuality: College Women's Gender Strategies and Homophobia." *Gender and Society* 21.2 (2007): 145–172.

Harris, Paul. "Metrosexual Man Bows to Red-Blooded Übersexuals." *TheGuardian.com.* Last modified October 23, 2005. http://www.theguardian.com/world/2005/oct/23/gender.books.

Harris-Lacewell, Melissa Victoria. *Barbershops, Bibles, and BET: Everyday Talk and Black Political Thought.* Princeton, NJ: Princeton University Press, 2010.

Harvey Wingfield, Adia. "Are Some Emotions Marked 'Whites Only'? Racialized Feeling Rules in Professional Workplaces." *Social Problems* 57.2 (2010): 251–268.

———. *Doing Business with Beauty: Black Women, Hair Salons, and the Racial Enclave Economy.* New York: Rowman and Littlefield, 2008.

———. *No More Invisible Man: Race and Gender in Men's Work.* Philadelphia: Temple University Press, 2013.

———. "Racializing the Glass Escalator: Reconsidering Men's Experiences with Women's Work." *Gender and Society* 23.1 (2009): 5–26.

Hays, Sharon. *The Cultural Contradictions of Motherhood.* New Haven, CT: Yale University Press, 1996.

———. "Structure and Agency and the Sticky Problem of Culture." *Sociological Theory* 12.1 (1994): 57–72.

Hesse-Biber, Sharlene Nagy, and Michelle L. Yaiser, eds. *Feminist Perspectives on Social Research.* Oxford: Oxford University Press, 2004.

Hochschild, Arlie. *The Managed Heart: Commercialization of Human Feeling.* Berkeley: University of California Press, 1983.

Hogan, William Ransom, and Edwin Adams Davis. *William Johnson's Natchez: The Ante-Bellum Diary of a Free Negro.* Baton Rouge: Louisiana State University Press, 1951.

Holland, Samantha. *Alternative Femininities: Body, Age, and Identity.* New York: Berg Publishers, 2004.

Hondagneu-Sotelo, Pierette. *Doméstica: Immigrant Workers Cleaning and Caring in the Shadows of Affluence.* Berkeley: University of California Press, 2001.

Hondagneu-Sotelo, Pierette, and Michael A. Messner. "Gender Displays and Men's Power: The 'New Man' and the Mexican Immigrant Man." In *Theorizing Masculinities*, edited by Harry Brod and Michael Kaufman, 200–218. Thousand Oaks, CA: Sage Publications, 1994.

Hoovers, A Dun and Bradstreet Company. *Supercuts, Inc.* Short Hills, NJ: Hoovers, A Dun and Bradstreet Company, 2009.

———. *Supercuts, Inc. Profile.* Austin, TX: Hoovers, A Dun and Bradstreet Company, 2015.

IBISWorld. *Hair and Nail Salons in the US—Industry Market Research Report.* Los Angeles: IBISWorld, August 2008.

———. *Hair and Nail Salons in the US—Industry Market Research Report.* Los Angeles: IBISWorld, August 2010.

———. *Hair Salons in the US—IBISWorld Industry Report 0D4410.* Los Angeles: IBISWorld, February 2015.

———. *Hair and Nail Salons in the US—IBISWorld Industry Report 81211.* Los Angeles: IBISWorld, February 2015.

Ingraham, Chrys. "The Heterosexual Imaginary: Feminist Sociology and Theories of Gender." *Sociological Theory* 12.2 (1994): 203–219.

Jacobs-Huey, Lanita. *From the Kitchen to the Parlor: Language and Becoming in African American Women's Hair Care.* New York: Oxford University Press, 2006.

Johnson, Steve. "Labels Come, Go, But Trendy Men Are Here to Shave." *Chicago Tribune,* July 28, 2004. http://articles.chicagotribune.com/2004-07-28/features/0407280033_1_metrosexual-hair-cuttery-sports-illustrated-swimsuit-issue.

Jones, Christian R. *Barbershop: History and Antiques.* Atglen, PA: Schiffer, 1999.

Kang, Miliann. "The Managed Hand: The Commercialization of Bodies and Emotions in Korean Immigrant-Owned Nail Salons." *Gender and Society* 17.6 (2003): 820–839.

———. *The Managed Hand: Race, Gender, and the Body in Beauty Service Work.* Berkeley: University of California Press, 2010.

Kanter, Rosabeth Moss. *Men and Women of the Corporation*. New York: Basic Books, 1977.

Kessler, Suzanne J., and Wendy McKenna. *Gender: An Ethnomethodological Approach.* Chicago: University of Chicago Press, 1985.

Kimmel, Michael. S. "Consuming Manhood: The Feminization of American Culture and the Recreation of the American Male Body, 1832–1920." *Michigan Quarterly Review* 33.1 (1994): 7–36.

———. "'Gender Symmetry' in Domestic Violence: A Substantive and Methodological Research Review." *Violence Against Women* 8.11 (2002): 1332–1363.

———. *Manhood in America: A Cultural History.* New York: The Free Press, 1996.

———. "Masculinity as Homophobia: Fear, Shame, and Silence in the Construction of Gender Identity." In *Theorizing Masculinities*, edited by Harry Brod and Michael Kaufman, 119–141. Thousand Oaks, CA: Sage, 1994.

———. "Men's Responses to Feminism at the Turn of the Century." *Gender and Society* 1.3 (1987): 261–283.

Kimmel, Michael S., and Abby L. Ferber, eds. *Privilege.* Boulder, CO: Westview Press, 2003.

Kirkham, Pat. *The Gendered Object.* Manchester, UK: Manchester University Press, 1996.

Klein, Alan M. *Little Big Men: Bodybuilding Subculture and Gender Construction.* Albany: State University of New York Press, 1993.

Kvande, Elin. "'In the Belly of the Beast': Constructing Femininities in Engineering Organizations." *European Journal of Women's Studies* 6.3 (1999): 305–328.

Kynaston, Lee. "Five Women's Beauty Products that Men Should 'Borrow.'" *The Telegraph*, October 11, 2013. http://www.telegraph.co.uk/men/fashion-and-style/10365171/ Five-womens-beauty-products-that-men-should-borrow.html.

Lareau, Annette. *Unequal Childhoods: Class, Race, and Family Life.* Berkeley: University of California Press, 2003.

Leidner, Robin. *Fast Food, Fast Talk: Service Work and the Routinization of Everyday Life.* Berkeley: University of California Press, 1993.

Levinson, Barry. "(How) Can a Man Do Feminist Ethnography of Education?" *Qualitative Inquiry* 4.3 (1998): 337–369.

Levy, Ariel. *Female Chauvinist Pigs: Women and the Rise of Raunch Culture.* New York: Free Press, 2005.

Lively, Kathryn J. "Reciprocal Emotion Management: Working Together to Maintain Stratification in Private Law Firms." *Work and Occupations* 27.1 (2000): 32–63.

London, Bianca. "Metrosexual Men Cost Their Partners £230 Every Year in Beauty Products . . . and It's All David Beckham's Fault." *MailOnline*, July 1, 2013. http:// www.dailymail.co.uk/femail/article-2352279/Metrosexual-men-cost-partners-230 -year-beauty-products-bid-look-groomed-like-David-Beckham.html.

Lorber, Judith. "Beyond the Binaries: Depolarizing the Categories of Sex, Sexuality, and Gender." *Sociological Inquiry* 66.2 (1996): 143–160.

———. *Breaking the Bowls: Degendering and Feminist Change.* New York: W.W. Norton, 2005.

———. *Paradoxes of Gender*. New Haven, CT: Yale University Press, 1994.

Luciano, Lynne. *Looking Good: Male Body Image in Modern America*. New York: Hill and Wang, 2001.

MacKinnon, Catherine A. *Sexual Harassment of Working Women*. New Haven, CT: Yale University Press, 1979.

Maines, Rachel P. *The Technology of Orgasm: "Hysteria," the Vibrator, and Women's Sexual Satisfaction*. Baltimore, MD: Johns Hopkins University Press, 1998.

Mardi Gras: Made in China. Directed by David Redmon. New York: Carnivalesque Films, 2008. DVD.

Martin, Patricia Yancey. "'Said and Done' vs. 'Saying and Doing': Gendering Practices, Practicing Gender at Work." *Gender and Society* 17.3 (2003): 342–366.

McCaughey, Martha. *The Caveman Mystique: Pop-Darwinism and the Debates Over Sex, Violence, and Science*. London: Routledge, 2008.

McCormack, Mark. "Hey, Bro, Let's Cuddle: Why the Modern Man Likes to Touch." *Playboy*, August 26, 2014. http://www.playboy.com/articles/why-modern-men -like-to-cuddle.

McDowell, Colin. *The Man of Fashion: Peacock Males and Perfect Gentlemen*. New York: Thames and Hudson, 1997.

McIntosh, Peggy. "White Privilege: Unpacking the Invisible Knapsack." *Peace and Freedom*, 1989. http://www.areteadventures.com/articles/white_privilege_unpacking _the_invisble_napsack.pdf.

McPherson, Miller, Lynn Smith-Lovin, and Matthew E. Brashears. "Social Isolation in America: Changes in Core Discussion Networks over Two Decades." *American Sociological Review* 71.3 (2006): 353–375.

Mead, George Herbert. *George Herbert Mead: On Social Psychology—Selected Papers*. Edited by Anselm Strauss. 1934. Reprint, Chicago: University of Chicago Press, 1964.

Merton, Robert K. "Insiders and Outsiders: A Chapter in the Sociology of Knowledge." *American Journal of Sociology* 78.1 (1972): 9–47.

Messerschmidt, James W. "Becoming 'Real Men.' Adolescent Masculinity Challenges and Sexual Violence." *Men and Masculinities* 2.3 (2000): 286–307.

———. *Nine Lives: Adolescent Masculinities, the Body, and Violence*. Boulder, CO: Westview Press, 2000.

Messner, Michael A. "Barbie Girls versus Sea Monsters: Children Constructing Gender." *Gender and Society* 14.6 (2000): 765–784.

———. *Power at Play: Sports and the Problem of Masculinity*. Boston: Beacon Press, 1992.

———. "Sports and Male Domination: The Female Athlete as Contested Ideological Terrain." *Sociology of Sport Journal* 5.3 (1988): 197–211.

———. "When Bodies Are Weapons: Masculinity and Violence in Sport." *International Review for the Sociology of Sport* 25.3 (1990): 203–220.

Messner, Michael A., Margaret Carlisle Duncan, and Kerry Jensen. "Separating the Men from the Girls: The Gendered Language of Television Sports." *Gender and Society* 7.1 (1993): 121–137.

Messner, Michael A., and Jeffrey Montez de Oca. "The Male Consumer as Loser: Beer and Liquor Ads in Mega Sports Media Events." *Signs: Journal of Women in Culture and Society* 30.3 (2005): 1879–1909.

Messner, Michael A., and Donald F. Sabo. *Sex, Violence, and Power in Sports: Rethinking Masculinity*. Freedom, CA: The Crossing Press, 1994.

Miller, Jody. *One of the Guys: Girls, Gangs, and Gender*. New York: Oxford University Press, 2001.

Miller, Laura. *Beauty Up: Exploring Contemporary Japanese Body Aesthetics*. Berkeley: University of California Press, 2006.

Mills, C. Wright. *White-Collar: The American Middle Class*. New York: Oxford University Press, 1951.

Morgan-Curtis, Samantha A. "Misogyny." In *International Encyclopedia of Men and Masculinities*, edited by Michael Flood, Judith Kegan Gardiner, Bob Pease, and Keith Pringle, 443–445. New York: Routledge, 2007.

Moskovic, Daniel J., Michael L. Eisenberg, and Larry I. Lipshultz. "Seasonal Fluctuations in Testosterone-Estrogen Ratio in Men from the Southwest United States." *Journal of Andrology* 33.6 (2012): 1298–1304.

Mukherjee, Roopali. "The Ghetto Fabulous Aesthetic in Contemporary Black Culture: Class and Consumption in the *Barbershop* Film." *Cultural Studies* 20.6 (2006): 599–629.

Munsch, Christin L. and Robb Willer. "The Role of Gender Identity Threat in Perceptions of Date Rape and Sexual Coercion." *Violence Against Women* 18.10 (2012): 1125–1146.

Murphy, Peter F. *Studs, Tools, and the Family Jewels*. Madison: University of Wisconsin Press, 2001.

Musso, Fabio, and Elena Druica. *Handbook of Research on Retailer-Consumer Relationship Development*. Hershey, PA: IGI Global, 2014.

NAILS Magazine. *2014–2015 Big Book: Everything You Need to Know About the Nail Industry*. Torrance, CA: Bobit Business Media, 2015. http://files.nailsmag.com/Market-Research/NABB2014–2015-Stats-2-1.pdf.

Naples, Nancy A. "A Feminist Revisiting of the Insider/Outsider Debate: The 'Outsider Phenomenon' in Rural Iowa." *Qualitative Sociology* 19.1 (1996): 83–106.

Novick, Gina. "Is There a Bias Against Telephone Interviews in Qualitative Research?" *Research in Nursing and Health* 31.4 (2008): 391–398.

Oakley, Ann. "Interviewing Women: A Contradiction in Terms?" In *Doing Feminist Research*, edited by Helen Roberts, 30–61. London: Routledge and Kegan Paul, 1981.

O'Brien, Glenn. "Male Facials." *GQ*, May 14, 2006, http://www.gq.com/style/style-guy/grooming/200605/facials-men.

———. "Manicures for Men?," *GQ*, July 8, 2009, http://www.gq.com/style/style-guy/grooming/200907/manicures-for-men.

O'Brien, Martin. "*The Managed Heart* Revisited: Health and Social Control." *Sociological Review* 42.3 (1994): 393–413.

Oerton, Sarah. "Bodywork Boundaries: Power, Politics, and Professionalism in Therapeutic Massage." *Gender, Work, and Organization* 11.5 (2004): 544–565.

Oerton, Sarah, and Joanne Phoenix. "Sex/Body Work: Discourses and Practices." *Sexualities* 4.4 (2001): 387–412.

Oldenburg, Ray. *Celebrating the Third Place: Inspiring Stories About the 'Great Good Places' at the Heart of Our Communities.* New York: Marlow & Co., 2001.

———. *The Great Good Place: Cafés, Coffee Shops, Community Centers, Beauty Parlors, General Stores, Bars, Hangouts, and How They Get You Through the Day.* New York: Paragon House, 1989.

Otis, Eileen M. "The Dignity of Working Women: Service, Sex, and the Labor Politics of Localization in China's City of Eternal Spring." *American Behavioral Scientist* 52.3 (2008): 356–376.

———. *Markets and Bodies: Women, Service Work, and the Making of Inequality in China.* Stanford, CA: Stanford University Press, 2011.

Paap, Kris. *Working Construction: Why White Working Class Men Put Themselves— and the Labor Movement—in Harm's Way.* Ithaca, NY: Cornell University Press, 2006.

Parreñas, Rhacel. "Hostess Work: Negotiating the Morals of Money and Sex." In *Economic Sociology of Work*, Vol. 19 of *Research in the Sociology of Work*, edited by Nina Bandelj, 201–232. Bingley, UK: Emerald, 2009.

Pascoe, C. J. *Dude, You're a Fag: Masculinity and Sexuality in High School.* Berkeley: University of California Press, 2007.

Peiss, Kathy. *Hope in a Jar: The Making of America's Beauty Culture.* New York: Henry Holt and Company, 1998.

Pettinger, Lynne. "Gendered Work Meets Gendered Goods: Selling and Service in Clothing Retail." *Gender, Work, and Organization* 12.5 (2005): 460–478.

Pierce, Jennifer L. *Gender Trials: Emotional Lives in Contemporary Law Firms.* Berkeley: University of California Press, 1996.

Poynton, Cate. *Language and Gender: Making the Difference.* Geelong, Australia: Deakin University Press, 1985.

Presser, Lois. "Negotiating Power and Narrative in Research: Implications for Feminist Methodology." *Signs: Journal of Women in Culture and Society* 30.4 (2005): 2067–2090.

"Pretty Handsome! More Men Buying Women's Beauty Products." *New York Daily News*, June 29, 2012. http://www.nydailynews.com/life-style/fashion/report-men-increasingly-buying-women-beauty-products-article-1.1104625.

Pyke, Karen D., and Denise L. Johnson. "Asian American Women and Radicalized Femininities: 'Doing' Gender across Cultural Worlds." *Gender and Society* 17.1 (2003): 33–53.

Quintanilla, Michael. "H-E-B Aisle Is for Guys Only." *Houston Chronicle*, January 27, 2010. http://www.chron.com/life/article/H-E-B-aisle-is-for-guys-only-1708148.php.

Ranson, Gillian. "No Longer 'One of the Boys': Negotiations with Motherhood, as Prospect or Reality, among Women in Engineering." *Canadian Review of Sociology* 42.2 (2005): 145–166.

Reindl, JC. "Hipster Barbershops: Young Men Seek Some Old-Fashioned Grooming." *Detroit Free Press*, February 20, 2015. http://www.gosanangelo.com/lifestyle/hipster-barbershops-young-men-seek-some-oldfashioned-grooming_19965231.

Rhoton, Laura. "Distancing as a Gendered Barrier: Understanding Women Scientists' Gender Practices." *Gender and Society* 25.6 (2011): 696–716.

Risman, Barbara J. "Gender as a Social Structure: Theory Wrestling with Activism." *Gender and Society* 18.4 (2004): 429–450.

Ritzer, George. *Explorations in the Sociology of Consumption: Fast Food Restaurants, Cards, and Casinos*, Vol. 2. London: Sage, 2001.

Rivas, Lynn May. "Invisible Labors: Caring for the Independent Person." In *Global Woman: Nannies, Maids, and Sex Workers in the New Economy*, edited by Barbara Ehrenreich and Arlie Russell Hochschild, 70–84. New York: Henry Holt and Company, 2002.

Roach, Joseph. *Cities of the Dead: Circum-Atlantic Performance*. New York: Columbia University Press, 1996.

Rolston, Jessica Smith. *Mining Coal and Undermining Gender: Rhythms of Work and Family in the American West*. New Brunswick, NJ: Rutgers University Press, 2014.

Roosters Men's Grooming Center, a Division of Regis Corporation. Minneapolis, MN: Regis Corporation. http://www.roostersmgc.com/Locations/.

Rosenberg, Karen. "An Art Trove Built on Mascara and Cold Cream: Celebrating Helena Rubinstein at the Jewish Museum." *New York Times*, October 30, 2014. http://www.nytimes.com/2014/10/31/arts/design/celebrating-helena-rubinstein-at-the-jewish-museum.html?_r=1.

Rubin, Gayle S. "Thinking Sex: Notes for a Radical Theory of the Politics of Sexuality." In *The Lesbian and Gay Studies Reader*, edited by Harry Abelove, Michele Aina Barale, and David M. Halperin, 3–44. New York: Routledge, 1984.

Rupp, Leila J. and Verta Taylor. *Drag Queens at the 801 Cabaret*. Chicago: University of Chicago Press, 2003.

Sanders, Teela. "Controllable Laughter: Managing Sex Work through Humour." *Sociology* 38.2 (2004): 273–291.

Sanders, Teela, Rachel Lara Cohen, and Kate Hardy. "Hairdressing/Undressing: Comparing Labour Relations in Self-Employed Body Work." In *Body/Sex/Work: Intimate, Embodied, and Sexualised Labour*, edited by Carol Wolkowitz, Rachel Lara Cohen, Teela Sanders, and Kate Hardy, 110–126. London: Palgrave Macmillan, 2013.

Schilt, Kristen. *Just One of the Guys? Transgender Men and the Persistence of Gender Inequality*. Chicago: University of Chicago Press, 2010.

Schippers, Mimi. "Recovering the Feminine Other: Masculinity, Femininity, and Gender Hegemony." *Theory and Society* 36.1 (2007): 85–102.

Schlossman, Fallon and Louisa Alter. "Trend Alert: Men, It's Okay to Care About Your Hair." *WNYC*, July 23, 2015. http://www.wnyc.org/story/trend-alert-its-okay-care/.

Schwalbe, Michael L. and Douglas Mason-Schrock. "Identity Work as Group Process." In *Advance in Group Processes*, Vol. 13, edited by Shane R. Thye and Edward J. Lawler, 115–149. Greenwich, CT: JAI Press, 1996.

Schwalbe, Michael L. and Michelle Wolkomir. "The Masculine Self as Problem and Resource in Interview Studies of Men." *Men and Masculinities* 4.1 (2001): 90–103.

Sharma, Ursula, and Paula Black. "Look Good, Feel Better: Beauty Therapy as Emotional Labour." *Sociology* 35.4 (2001): 913–931.

Sherman, Rachel. *Class Acts: Service and Inequality in Luxury Hotels*. Berkeley: University of California Press, 2007.

Shuy, Roger. *Linguistic Battles in Trademark Disputes*. New York: Macmillan, 2002.

Simpson, Mark. "Ryan Lochte Manscapes for Hours—With Liberace's Razors." *MarkSimpson.com*. Last modified May 3, 2013. http://www.marksimpson.com/blog/2013/05/03/ryan-lochte-manscapes-for-hours-with-liberaces-razors/.

Smith, Dorothy E. "Women's Perspectives as a Radical Critique of Sociology." In *Feminism and Methodology: Social Science Issues*, edited by Sandra Harding, 84–96. Bloomington: Indiana University Press, 2004.

Smith, Kristin. "Recessions Accelerate Trend of Wives as Breadwinners." *Carsey School of Public Policy at the Scholars' Repository*, 2012. http://scholars.unh.edu/carsey/181.

Stacey, Judith. "Can There Be a Feminist Ethnography?" *Women's Studies International Forum* 11.1 (1988): 21–27.

Stanley, Liz, and Sue Wise. *Breaking Out: Feminist Consciousness and Feminist Research*. London: Routledge and Kegan Paul, 1983.

Stephens, Neil. "Collecting Data from Elites and Ultra Elites: Telephone and Face-to-Face Interviews with Macroeconomists." *Qualitative Research* 7.2 (2007): 203–216.

St. John, Warren. "Metrosexuals Come Out." *New York Times*, June 22, 2003. http://www.nytimes.com/2003/06/22/style/metrosexuals-come-out.html.

Stone, Pamela. *Opting Out?: Why Women Really Quit Careers and Head Home*. Berkeley: University of California Press, 2007.

Tamayo, Yvonne A. "Rhymes with Rich: Power, Law, and the Bitch." *St. Thomas Law Review* 21.3 (2009): 281–301.

Taylor, Catherine J. "Physiological Stress Response to Loss of Social Influence and Threats to Masculinity." *Social Science and Medicine* 103 (2014): 51–59.

Taylor, Steve, and Melissa Tyler. "Emotional Labour and Sexual Difference in the Airline Industry." *Work, Employment & Society* 14.1 (2000): 77–95.

Taylor, Verta, and Leila J. Rupp. "When the Girls Are Men: Negotiating Gender and Sexual Dynamics in a Study of Drag Queens." *Signs: Journal of Women in Culture and Society* 30.4 (2005): 2115–2139.

Thomas, Arthur E. "Future Shock from a Black Perspective." *Theory into Practice* 20.4 (1981): 237–244.

Thorne, Barrie. *Gender Play: Girls and Boys in School*. New Brunswick, NJ: Rutgers University Press, 1993.

Traister, Aaron. "'Retrosexuals': The Latest Lame Macho Catchphrase." *Salon.com*. Last modified April 7, 2010. http://www.salon.com/2010/04/07/retrosexuals_silliness/.

Trautner, Mary Nell. "Doing Gender, Doing Class: The Performance of Sexuality in Exotic Dance Clubs." *Gender and Society* 19.6 (2005): 771–788.

Tungate, Mark. *Branded Beauty: How Marketing Changed the Way We Look*. London: Kogan Page, 2011.

United States Census Bureau, County Business Patterns. "Data Tables by Enterprise Receipt Size: U.S., All Industries." Washington, DC: U.S. Census Bureau, 2015. https://www.census.gov/econ/susb/.

U.S. Department of Commerce, Economics and Statistics Administration. "Census of Service Industries: Sources of Receipts of Revenue." Washington, DC: Bureau of the Census, 1992.

U.S. Department of Labor, Bureau of Labor Statistics. "Databases, Tables and Calculators by Subject: Los Angeles–Long Beach–Anaheim, CA Metropolitan Statistical Area Unemployment Rate." Washington, DC: Bureau of Labor Statistics, 2015.

———. "Household Data Annual Averages: Employed Persons by Detailed Occupation, Sex, Race, and Hispanic or Latino Ethnicity." Washington, DC: Bureau of Labor Statistics, 2015.

———. "Household Data Annual Averages: Employed Status of the Civilian Noninstitutional Population, 1944 to Date." Washington, DC: Bureau of Labor Statistics, 2015.

———. "Occupational Employment and Wages: Barbers." Washington, DC: Bureau of Labor Statistics, 2014.

———. "Occupational Employment and Wages: Hairdressers, Hairstylists, and Cosmetologists." Washington, DC: Bureau of Labor Statistics, 2014.

Wade, Lisa. "American Men's Hidden Crisis: They Need More Friends!" *Salon*, December 7, 2013. http://www.salon.com/2013/12/08/american_mens_hidden_crisis_they_need_more_friends/.

Warhurst, Chris, and Dennis Nickson. "Employee Experience of Aesthetic Labour in Retail and Hospitality." *Work, Employment, and Society* 21.1 (2007): 103–120.

———. "'Who's Got the Look?' Emotional, Aesthetic, and Sexualized Labour in Interactive Services." *Gender, Work, and Organization* 16.3 (2009): 385–404.

Wax, Rosaline H. "Gender and Age in Fieldwork and Fieldwork Education: 'Not Any Good Thing Is Done by One Man Alone.'" In *Self, Sex, and Gender in Cross-Cultural Fieldwork*, edited by Tony L. Whitehead and Mary E. Conaway, 129–150. 1970. Reprint. Chicago: University of Illinois Press, 1986.

Weitz, Rose. *Rapunzel's Daughters: What Women's Hair Tells Us about Women's Lives.* New York: Farrar, Straus and Giroux, 2004.

Wenner, Lawrence A. "In Search of the Sports Bar: Masculinity, Alcohol, Sports, and the Mediation of Public Space." In *Sport and Postmodern Times*, edited by Genevieve Rail, 301–332. Albany: State University of New York Press, 1998.

West, Candace, and Sarah Fenstermaker. "Doing Difference." *Gender and Society* 9.1 (1995): 8–37.

West, Candace, and Don H. Zimmerman. "Doing Gender." *Gender and Society* 1.2 (1987): 125–151.

Wier, Sadye H., and John F. Marszalek. *A Black Businessman in White Mississippi, 1886–1974.* Jackson: University of Mississippi Press, 1977.

Willer, Robb, Bridget Conlon, Christabel L. Rogalin, and Michael T. Wojnowicz. "Overdoing Gender: A Test of the Masculine Overcompensation Thesis." *American Journal of Sociology* 118.4 (2013): 980–1022.

Willett, Julia A. *Permanent Waves: The Making of the American Beauty Shop.* New York: New York University Press, 2000.

Williams, Alex. "Glenn O'Brien Reinvents Himself (Yet Again)." *The New York Times*, November 11, 2015. http://www.nytimes.com/2015/11/12/fashion/glenn-obrien -reinvents-himself-yet-again.html?_r=0.

Williams, Christine L. "The Glass Escalator: Hidden Advantages for Men in the 'Female' Professions." *Social Problems* 39.3 (1992): 253–267.

———. *Inside Toyland: Working, Shopping, and Social Inequality.* Berkeley: University of California Press, 2006.

Williams, Christine L., and Catherine Connell. "'Looking Good and Sounding Right': Aesthetic Labor and Social Inequality in the Retail Industry." *Work and Occupations* 37.3 (2010): 349–377.

Williams, Christine L., Patti A. Giuffre, and Kirsten Dellinger. "The Gay-Friendly Closet." *Sexuality Research and Social Policy: Journal of NSRC* 6.1 (2009): 29–45.

———. "Sexuality in the Workplace: Organizational Control, Sexual Harassment, and the Pursuit of Pleasure." *Annual Review of Sociology* 25.1 (1999): 73–93.

Williams, Christine L., and E. Joel Heikes. "The Importance of Researcher's Gender in the In-Depth Interview: Evidence from Two Case Studies of Male Nurses." *Gender and Society* 7.2 (1993): 280–291.

Williams, Claire. "Sky Service: The Demands of Emotional Labour in the Airline Industry." *Gender, Work, and Organization* 10.5 (2003): 513–550.

Williams, Louis. "The Relationship between a Black Barbershop and the Community That Supports It." *Human Mosaic* 27.1–2 (1993): 29–33.

Witz, Anne, Chris Warhurst, and Dennis Nickson. "The Labour of Aesthetics and the Aesthetics of Organization." *Organization* 10.1 (2003): 33–54.

Wolf, Diane L. "Situating Feminist Dilemmas in Fieldwork." In *Feminist Dilemmas in Fieldwork*, edited by Diane L. Wolf, 1–55. Boulder, CO: Westview Press, 1996.

Wolf, Naomi. *The Beauty Myth: How Images of Beauty Are Used against Women.* New York: Random House, 1991.

Wolkowitz, Carol. *Bodies at Work.* Thousand Oaks, CA: Sage Publications, 2006.

Women's Health Program, Monash University. "Testosterone and Androgens in Women." Last modified October 2010. http://med.monash.edu.au/sphspm/ womenshealth/docs/testosterone-and-androgens-in-women.pdf.

Wright, Earl II. "More Than Just a Haircut: Sociability within the Urban African American Barbershop." *Challenge: A Journal of Research on African American Men* 9 (1998): 1–13.

Wright, Earl II, and Thomas C. Calhoun. "From the Common Thug to the Local Businessman: An Exploration into an Urban African American Barbershop." *Deviant Behavior: An Interdisciplinary Journal* 22.3 (2001): 267–288.

Xie, Yu, and Kimberlee A. Shauman. *Women in Science: Career Processes and Outcomes.* Cambridge, MA: Harvard University Press, 2003.

Yeadon-Lee, Tracey. "Doing Identity with Style: Service Interaction, Work Practices, and the Construction of 'Expert' Status in the Contemporary Hair Salon." *Sociological Research Online* 17.4 (2012). doi: 10.5153/sro.2726

Yount, Kristen. "Ladies, Flirts and Tomboys: Strategies for Managing Sexual Harassment in an Underground Coal Mine." *Journal of Contemporary Ethnography* 19.4 (1991): 396–422.

Zelizer, Viviana A. *The Purchase of Intimacy*. Princeton, NJ: Princeton University Press, 2007.

Zerubavel, Eviatar. "Islands of Meaning." In *The Production of Reality: Essays and Readings on Social Interaction*, 5th ed., edited by Jodi A. O'Brien, 11–27. 1991. Reprint, Thousand Oaks, CA: Sage Publications, 2011.

Zimmerman, Gregory M., and Steven Messner. "Neighborhood Context and the Gender Gap in Adolescent Violent Crime." *American Sociological Review* 75.6 (2010): 958–980.

INDEX

acculturation, 51

Acker, Joan, 60, 109

Adkins, Lisa, 78

aesthetic: agency, 79; care, 67; classed, 93; enhancement, 161, 171; feminine, 26; labor, 10–11, 19, 77–81, 84–85, 89–92, 103, 117, 141, 165–167; masculine, 1, 54, 71, 74; professional, 54, 74; sexual, 59; spatial markers, 58; superiority, 25; taste, 71. *See also* heterosexual aesthetic labor

African American. *See* black

Afros, 37–38. *See also* black: natural hair

agency: aesthetic, 79; financial, 32; in marginalized locations, 179; resistant, 168; for women, 101, 103

aggression, heterosexual, 61, 85, 88, 96, 100, 115. *See also* caveman mystique

American Revolution, 24

Arden, Elizabeth, 30

Ayer, Harriet Hubbard, 34

baldness, xi, 1, 22, 37, 71, 111, 161, 177. *See also* comb-over; Rogaine

barbers: black, 17, 70, 131; boycotting salons, 38; as men, 127, 131, 166; and the risk of feminization, 124; in salon ads, 82; supporting beauticians, 33, 169; and touch, 106

barbershops: black, 3, 42, 58, 71, 131, 166, 195n89; blue-collar, 114, 166; hipster, 58, 125, 166, 187n16; Latino, 42, 166; white, 14, 33, 37–38, 42–43, 58, 121, 166, 172

beautifying man, x, 7, 50, 55, 75

beauty: consumption of, x, 13, 18, 21, 23, 34, 41, 47, 69, 163, 166, 190n43, 208n10; culture, 4, 12, 18, 29, 31, 51, 65, 154, 156, 158, 168; educating men on, xi, 19, 69–71, 73–74, 129, 156 (*see also* initiating men into beauty); experts, 74, 155–156,

211n38; habits, of men, x, 2, 17, 45; language of, 51, 61; norms of, 5–6; politics of, xii, 24; practices, 7, 12, 57, 115, 129; products, x, 2, 21, 32–33, 39, 44–47, 73, 164; regimens, 1–2, 18, 24, 115; rhetoric of, 21, 162; spaces, 4, 18, 43, 46; terminology of, 19, 63–64; trends, 11. *See also* grooming

beauty business, 28–29, 31, 34, 38, 44–45; agents, 32; companies, male-owned, 36; entrepreneurs, 23, 29–32, 34–35, 169; industry, ix–xi, 2–4, 8, 11–12, 18–19, 21, 23, 29, 33–35, 41, 43–44, 66–77, 71, 74, 85, 123, 134, 161–162, 164, 177; shops, 6, 48–49, 62, 74, 121, 132

beauty colleges, 32–33

beauty workers: history of, 33; labor movement, 168–169; policy changes for, 21; relationships with each other, 151, 160; training, 32, 47, 63, 66, 70, 115, 115, 122, 138, 177

beer: advertisements, 40, 59; drinking, 57, 59–61, 163; serving, 9, 19, 48–49, 55, 59, 86, 89, 136, 147, 150, 154–155, 165; as a symbolic marker, 51, 59, 75

biological: difference, 73, 112; inclinations, 97–99, 108, 131, 167, 203n47; reality, 79; rhetoric, 72, 199n40. *See also* essentialism

Bird, Sharon, 54

"bitches," 133, 143, 160

black: barbers, 17, 70, 131; barbershops, 3, 42, 58, 71, 131, 166, 195n89; beauty, 29, 31, 37; beauty business, 31; cosmetic company, 35; entrepreneurs, 31, 116; natural hair, 37; neighborhoods, 58; stylists, 17; women, 6, 31, 33–34, 160, 166. *See also* men: of color; women: of color

ABOUT THE AUTHOR

KRISTEN BARBER is an assistant professor of sociology and a faculty affiliate in the Women, Gender, and Sexuality Studies Department at Southern Illinois University, Carbondale.